Colour **Aids**

Gastroenterology and Liver Disease

Gregory Holdstock DM MRCP

Consultant Physician,
Mount Vernon and Hillingdon Hospitals,
Middlesex, UK

Ralph Wright MA MD DPhil FRCP

Professor of Medicine,
University of Southampton, UK

D1412340

Churchill Livingstone

EDINBURGH LONDON MELBOURNE AND NEW YORK 1989

Acknowledgements

We would like to thank all those friends and colleagues who generously allowed us to borrow their slides. In particular we would like to thank Dr C.L. Smith, Dr J. Bamforth, Dr F. Burrows, Dr K. Dewberry, Dr Claire Duboulay, Dr H. Milward—Sadler and Dr Brian Cooper. We are also grateful to Dr Peter Hayes of the Royal Infirmary, Edinburgh, and Dr Margaret MacIntyre and the GI Unit at the Western General Hospital, Edinburgh, for the loan of Figures 47, 48, 57, 96, 97 and 113.

Contents

Gastroenterology

1 | The Mouth

Examination of the mouth may give useful clinical information.

Salivary glands

The salivary glands may be enlarged by tumour, infiltration or in systemic disease, including chronic liver disease and sarcoidosis.

Mouth

Aphthous ulcers may be found in coeliac disease or inflammatory bowel disease. Angular stomatitis and a smooth shiny tongue may be seen in deficiency states. The mouth may contract in systemic sclerosis.

Tongue

The tongue may be large as in amyloid. A white coating can be seen in candidiasis. A geographic tongue may be seen during ill-health.

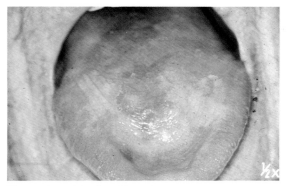

Fig. 1 Atrophic glossitis with angular stomatitis.

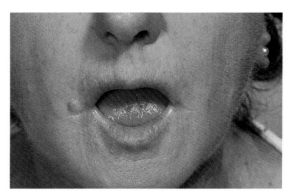

Fig. 2 The face in scleroderma showing contracture of mouth.

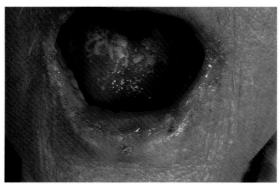

Fig. 3 Oral candidiasis.

2 | General Examination

General examination may reveal clues to underlying gastrointestinal malignancies.

Skin

Changes associated with occult GI malignancies, include dermatomyositis, acanthosis, tylosis and rapid onset of senile keratosis. There may be evidence of fistula formation.

Nails

The nails may show changes of systemic sclerosis, vasculitis, clubbing or features of chronic liver disease. Koilonychia is seen in longstanding iron deficiency anaemia.

Lymph glands

Generalised lymphadenopathy may be seen in neoplastic disease including lymphoma.

Legs

Thrombophlebitis is a rare presentation of pancreatic neoplasm and is often migratory.

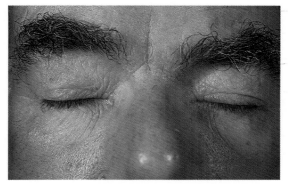

Fig. 4 Heliotrope discoloration in dermatomyositis.

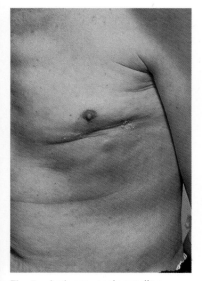

Fig. 5 Actinomycosis eroding through chest wall.

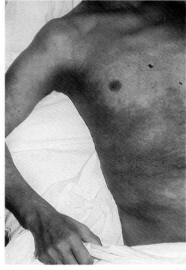

Fig. 6 Acanthosis nigricans.

3 | Oesophageal Webs and Rings

Definition

An oesophageal web is a stricture consisting of squamous mucosa. An oesophageal ring (Schatzki ring) marks the junction of oesophageal and gastric mucosa.

Symptoms

Usually present with intermittent dysphagia. Upper oesophageal web associated with iron deficiency anaemia is usually only found in women (Plummer–Vinson or Patterson Brown Kelly syndrome). An oesophageal ring may result in complete obstruction usually with meat bolus.

Treatment

Dilatation. Webs are easily broken with an endoscope.

Comment

Some authors doubt the significance of Schatzki rings and attribute symptoms to coexistent reflux.

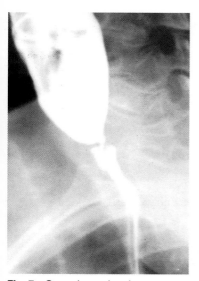

Fig. 7 Oesophageal web.

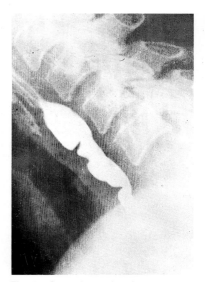

Fig. 8 Oesophageal web.

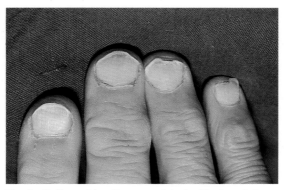

Fig. 9 Koilonychia often associated with chronic iron deficiency anaemia.

4 | Pharyngeal Pouch (Zenker's Diverticulum)

Definition

An outpouching of one or more layers of the oesophagus occurring immediately above the upper oesophageal sphincter. It probably results from a rise in pharyngeal pressure secondary to muscular discoordination.

Symptoms

Transient dysphagia, swelling in neck after eating, gurgling in throat with regurgitation of food shortly after swallowing. It can lead to pulmonary aspiration.

Diagnosis and Treatment

Best diagnosed radiologically since it can be perforated at endoscopy. If symptoms are sufficiently severe then it can be excised but an operation should be combined with cricopharyngeal myotomy to prevent recurrence.

Comment

The diverticulum can become very large. Diverticula also occur in the mid-oesophagus and above the lower oesophageal sphincter but these are rarely symptomatic.

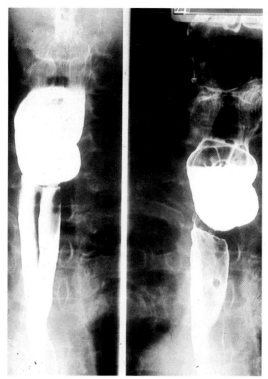

Fig. 10 Zenker's diverticulum.

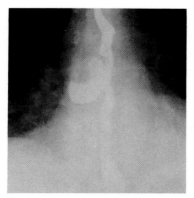

Fig. 11 Oesophageal pouch.

5 | Hiatus Hernia

Definition

Herniation of a portion of the stomach into the chest through the oesophageal hiatus of the diaphragm. Usually classified as (1) rolling when the gastric cardia rolls through the hiatus beside the OG junction which remains in the abdominal cavity and (2) sliding where both the stomach and the OG junction slip into the chest placing the OG junction above the diaphragmatic hernia, and (3) mixed. All may be intermittent or fixed.

Symptoms

Often asymptomatic and symptoms when present usually those of reflux. Rarely, it can incarcerate and present as a surgical emergency.

Barrett's oesophagus

Definition

Replacement of squamous epithelium by columnar epithelium. Usually occurs secondary to severe reflux oesophagitis.

Symptoms

Those of reflux oesophagitis. About 10% will develop oesophageal carcinoma and therefore should be regularly endoscoped to look for early changes. Aggressive anti-reflux measures may lead to regression of the disease.

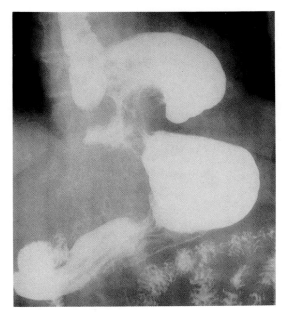

Fig. 12 Rolling hiatus hernia.

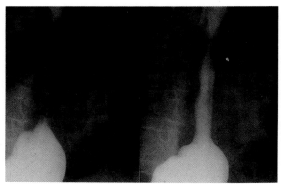

Fig. 13 Sliding hiatus hernia.

6 | Oesophageal Reflux (Reflux Oesophagitis)

Definition

Inflammation of oesophageal mucosa caused by reflux of acid or alkaline gastric contents.

Symptoms

Heartburn and dysphagia are often longstanding and related to posture (bending or lying flat).

Treatment

Dieting, avoid intra-abdominal pressure, advice regarding posture, avoid bending, elevate the head of the bed and simple antacids. If nocturnal symptoms are a problem avoid eating late at night. H_2 antagonists are useful if symptoms persist. Occasionally surgery may be necessary to repair hiatus and prevent reflux.

Diagnosis

Radiology may demonstrate reflux, often with hiatus hernia, but endoscopy with biopsy can confirm the presence of oesophagitis.

Comment

Rare complications include haemorrhage, oesophageal ulcer or stricture formation. Strictures can be treated by dilatation using progressively larger bougies (usually performed endoscopically).

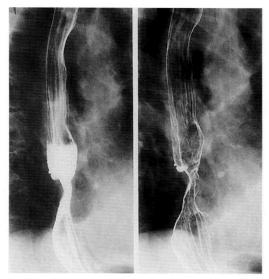

Fig. 14 Benign oesophageal stricture with reflux oesophagitis.

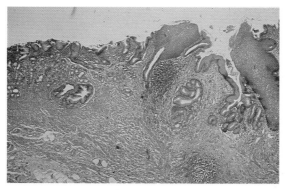

Fig. 15 Histology of Barrett's oesophagus.

7 | Oesophageal Motility Disorders

Definition

Disorders of oesophageal motility may result from increasing age (Presby oesophagus) or ganglion degeneration (as seen in achalasia).

Symptoms

Symptoms include dysphagia, regurgitation and chest pain which may be made worse by coexisting oesophagitis.

Diagnosis

Plain X-ray may reveal dilated oesophagus with fluid levels and absent gastric air bubble. Barium swallow shows abnormal motility with, in achalasia, a beak-like narrowing of the distal oesophagus (rat tail appearance). Typically, there is no resistance to the passage of an endoscope. Manometry shows high lower oesophageal sphincter pressure with failure to relax on swallowing.

Treatment

Coexisting reflux oesophagitis should be aggressively treated. Medical treatment with oral nitrates is of limited value. Achalasia can be dilated with a pneumatic dilator but disease invariably recurs. More permanent results can be obtained by splitting the cardiac sphincter surgically (Heller's operation).

Comment

Oesophageal spasm can be difficult to treat but it is important to recognise in order to avoid unnecessary cardiac investigation.

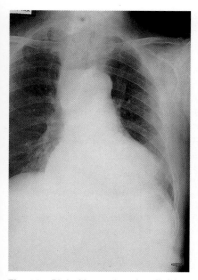

Fig. 16 Plain X-ray showing fluid level in dilated oesophagus with absent gastric bubble (achalasia).

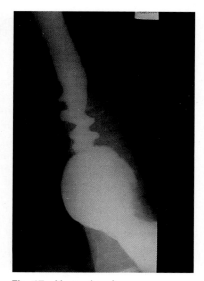

Fig. 17 X-ray showing severe oesophageal contractions and abnormal motility.

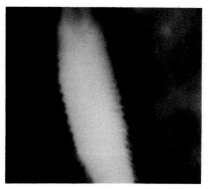

Fig. 18 Abnormal oesophageal motility.

8 | Oesophageal Cancer

Definition

Squamous cell carcinoma originating from oesophageal mucosa. Adenocarcinoma at lower end of oesophagus should be considered to be gastric in origin.

Epidemiology

Most common in men. Wide geographical variation in incidence, highest in north China and areas of Iran and the Soviet Union. Predisposing factors include smoking and longstanding chronic inflammation, particularly in Barrett's oesophagus. It also occurs in achalasia and tylosis, a rare familial condition of dyskeratosis of the soles of the feet and hands.

Symptoms

Progressive dysphagia, initially for solid food. Anaemia and systemic symptoms occur later.

Treatment

Surgical removal is the only method of cure but results are poor. Chemotherapy is not of proven value. Palliation can be achieved by insertion of a plastic tube through stricture, either endoscopically or surgically. Radiotherapy may give temporary relief for squamous tumours.

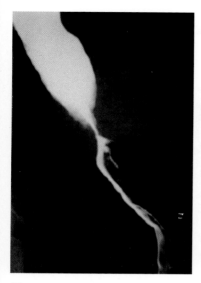

Fig. 19 Barium swallow showing a carcinoma of the oesophagus.

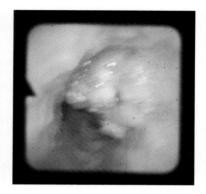

Fig. 20 Endoscopy view of oesophageal carcinoma.

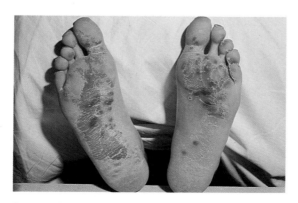

Fig. 21 Skin changes in tylosis associated with oesophageal cancer.

9 | Other Oesophageal Diseases

Ingestion of corrosives
Acute oesophagitis can result from ingestion of corrosives which may result in stricture formation.

Systemic disease
The oesophagus may be involved in systemic disease, especially systemic sclerosis.

Candidiasis
In immunocompromised hosts candida oesophagitis or herpes oesophagitis may occur and can be diagnosed by endoscopy and biopsy.

Chagas' disease
Chagas' disease (due to *Trypanosoma cruzi*), is a common cause of oesophageal disease in endemic areas and results from degeneration of intramural nerve plexus. It is confined to central and southern America.

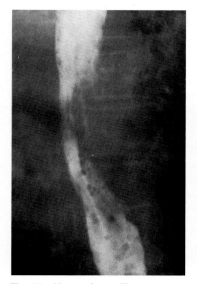

Fig. 22 X-ray of monilia oesophagitis.

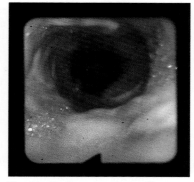

Fig. 23 Endoscopy of monilia oesophagitis.

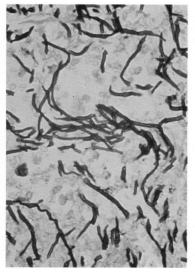

Fig. 24 Candidiasis on biopsy.

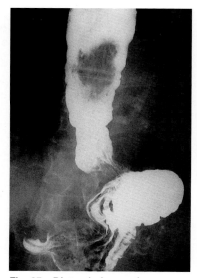

Fig. 25 Distended oesophagus with food debris in scleroderma.

10 | Peptic Ulcer Disease (1)

Definition

A breach in the gastric or duodenal mucosa. The depth of penetration varies. It may be acute or chronic. Gastric ulcers (GU) are commonly found on the lesser curve, posterior aspect or in antrum of the stomach. Duodenal ulcers (DU) are usually in the first or second parts of the duodenum.

Patho-physiology

It results from an imbalance between attacking (acid, pepsin and bile) and defending forces (mucus and cytoprojection of mucosa). Environmental, hereditary and psychic factors probably influence balance. Acid output tends to be normal or increased in DUs and normal or reduced in GUs. GUs and DUs should probably be considered as separate conditions.

Aetiology

They are more common in the lower social classes. Unknown dietary and genetic factors may be involved and both are more common in smokers. They are more often seen in patients with blood group O, particularly non-secretors. Drugs such as non-steroidal anti-inflammatory drugs and corticosteroids are occasionally involved in the pathogenesis.

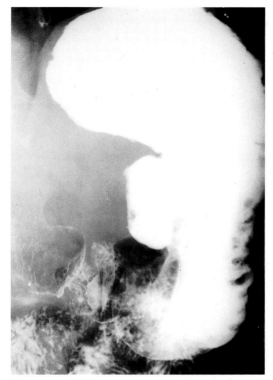

Fig. 26 Large gastric ulcer on lesser curve.

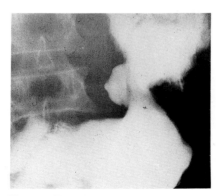

Fig. 27 Hourglass stomach associated with longstanding gastric ulcer.

10 | Peptic Ulcer (2)

Symptoms

Periodic epigastric pain related to meals and relieved by antacids. Anorexia, vomiting and weight loss may occur. The patient may present with the complication of haemorrhage or perforation or gastic outflow obstruction. Symptoms may be very varied and difficult to distinguish from those of gastric cancer, gall bladder or pancreatic disease. Similar symptoms may occur in patients with no demonstrable pathology (non-ulcer dyspepsia).

Diagnosis

There are no helpful features on examination. Often it is first diagnosed on barium meal but is best confirmed by endoscopy. Gastric ulcers need to be biopsied to exclude the possibility of malignancy.

Treatment

Antacids, and H_2 antagonists, e.g. cimetidine and ranitidine, form the mainstay of treatment. Other drugs aimed at increasing cytoprotection, such as Bismuth salts, Carbenoxolone, Sucralfate and Prostaglandin analogues, are second-line drugs. Surgery is required for resistant cases and for complications.

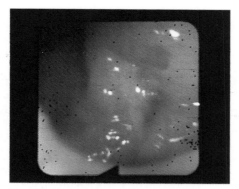

Fig. 28 Endoscopic view of gastric ulcer.

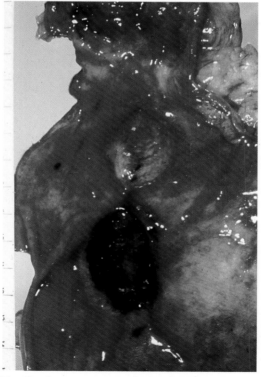

Fig. 29 Gastrectomy specimen of gastric ulcer.

Comment

Zollinger–Ellison syndrome should be considered when there are multiple duodenal ulcers present. Curling's ulcer occurs in patients with acute burns and Cushing's ulcer in those with mid-brain disease. Peptic ulcers are also found in the oesophagus when associated with reflux and occasionally in Meckel's diverticulum.

Zollinger–Ellison syndrome

Definition

A syndrome of multiple duodenal ulcers due to gastrin-secreting tumour usually, but not always, in the pancreas. It may be benign or malignant.

Symptoms

The symptoms are those of persistent duodenal ulcer disease and are often multiple. Diarrhoea and B_{12} deficiency are relatively common.

Treatment

The symptoms can normally be controlled by H_2 antagonists. If possible, laparotomy with highly selective vagotomy and resection of the tumour may be curative.

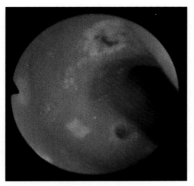

Fig. 30 Endoscopic view of duodenal ulcers.

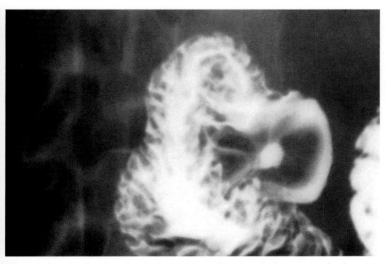

Fig. 31 X-ray of a duodenal ulcer with oedema and ulcer crater in the centre.

11 | Gastric Cancer

Definition

Adenocarcinoma originating from gastric mucosa.

Epidemiology

More common in men. Unknown environmental and genetic factors may be important. There is increased incidence in pernicious anaemia, following gastrectomy and in the syndrome of multiple gastric polyposis.

Symptoms

Progressive dyspepsia, abdominal pain, anorexia, vomiting and weight loss are most common. Also, iron deficiency anaemia or acute haemorrhage. Gastric outflow obstruction may occur—a succusion splash may then be heard.

Diagnosis

There may be an abdominal mass or evidence of liver metastases. Occasionally, a gland is palpable in the left supraclavicular region (Virchow's node). It can be diagnosed by barium meal but endoscopy and biopsy are preferable.

Treatment

Surgical or palliative.

Prognosis

Very poor with less than 5% five year survival except in the case of early gastric cancer, (disease confined to mucosa or submucosa where the prognosis is good). Chemotherapy and radiotherapy are of no proven benefit.

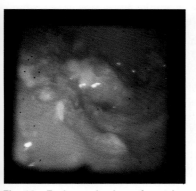

Fig. 32 Endoscopic view of gastric cancer.

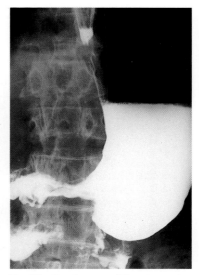

Fig. 33 Carcinoma of the stomach leading to pyloric outflow obstruction.

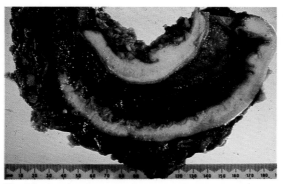

Fig. 34 Leather bottom stomach due to diffuse infiltrating gastric carcinoma.

12 | Gastric Polyps

Definition

Polyps originating in the gastric mucosa. They may be single or multiple. Most are regenerative but a few are adenomatous.

Symptoms

They are probably asymptomatic but occasionally can be seen in patients with dyspepsia.

Comment

Regenerative polyps can be left untreated. Because of malignant potential adenomatous ones should probably be removed either endoscopically or surgically especially when multiple.

Other Gastric Lesions

Leiomyoma
A benign tumour of the stomach which may be complicated by bleeding or malignancy.

Trichobezoar
A collection of hair or fibrous tissue usually seen in emotionally disturbed patients.

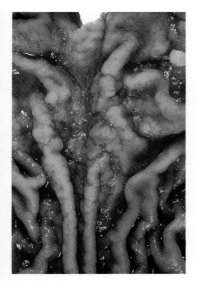

Fig. 35 Surgical specimen of multiple gastric polyps.

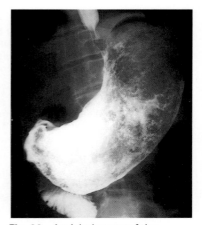

Fig. 36 A trichobezoar of the stomach on barium meal.

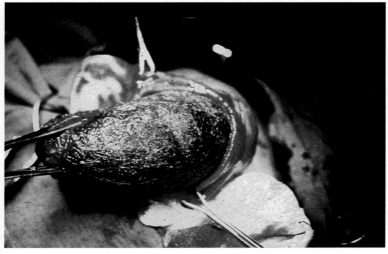

Fig. 37 A trichobezoar of the stomach being surgically removed.

13 | Gastritis

Definition

Inflammation of gastric mucosa. It may be acute, chronic, atrophic or hypertrophic. Hypertrophic gastritis should be considered as a separate entity (Menetrier's disease).

Patho-physiology

Very common, with increasing incidence related to advancing age. Cause is unknown but it is more common in smokers. Rarely it is associated with intrinsic factor deficiency (pernicious anaemia). *Campylobacter pylorii* is now suspected to be an important aetiological factor.

Symptoms

Unless complicated by some other process (such as peptic ulceration) it is probably not a cause of symptoms and is of unknown significance.

Comment

When severe and atrophic it may show features of intestinal metaplasia which may be a premalignant condition.

Duodenitis

Definition

Acute or chronic inflammation of duodenal mucosa.

Comment

Frequently seen in patients with duodenal ulcer in which the ulcer has healed. Relation to symptoms is unclear but it may be part of a duodenal ulcer diathesis.

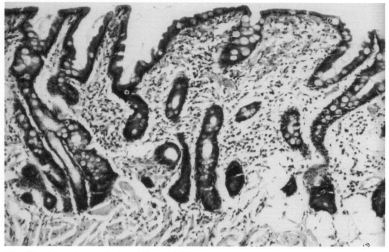

Fig. 38 Histology of atrophic gastritis.

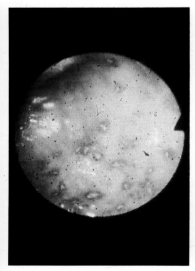

Fig. 39 Endoscopic view of gastritis.

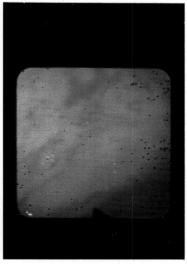

Fig. 40 Endoscopic view of Henoch–Schönlein syndrome affecting the stomach.

14 | Gastrointestinal Haemorrhage (1)

Definition

Bleeding into the GI tract. It may be acute and in severe cases present with shock; chronic cases present with iron deficiency anaemia.

Causes

1. *Upper tract.* Acute or chronic peptic ulcer, erosive gastritis, varices due to portal hypertension, oesophageal tear due to severe retching (Mallory–Weiss syndrome) and carcinoma of the stomach. Less commonly caused by oesophagitis, other neoplasms, vascular abnormalities (particularly hereditary haemorrhagic telangiectasia), bleeding into the biliary system (haematobilia) and the Peutz–Jeghers syndrome.
2. *Lower tract.* Diverticular disease, carcinoma of the colon or rectum, angiodysplasia, inflammatory bowel disease, colonic polyps and haemorrhoids. Also seen in radiation or ischaemic colitis, infective diarrhoea and infestations.

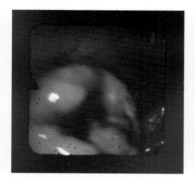

Fig. 41 Endoscopic view of leiomyoma of stomach with fresh bleeding.

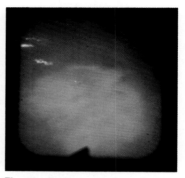

Fig. 42 Endoscopic view of acute haemorrhaging gastric erosions.

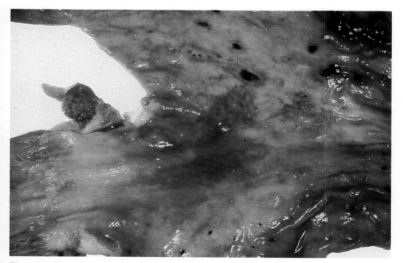

Fig. 43 Pathological specimen of acute gastric erosion.

14 | Gastrointestinal Haemorrhage (2)

Comment

Upper GI haemorrhage often presents with haematemesis which may be bright red or 'coffee-ground'. A history of retching prior to haematemesis should suggest diagnosis of Mallory–Weiss tear. A history of alcohol or aspirin ingestion prior to the episode suggests erosive gastritis. Lower GI haemorrhage may present occultly, with melaena suggesting a right-sided cause, or with bright red blood. Blood in the toilet pan and on paper suggests anal or low rectal cause. In all but young patients blood loss should not be attributed to haemorrhoids without examination of the colon. Meckel's diverticulum and small bowel tumours may also present with GI blood loss and should be considered when no other cause is found.

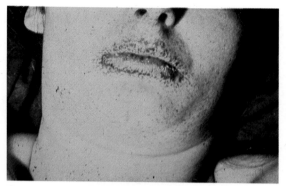

Fig. 44 The mouth in Peutz–Jeghers syndrome.

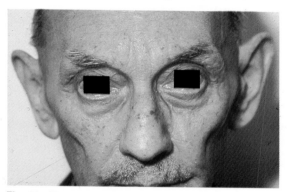

Fig. 45 The face in congenital haemorrhagic telangiectasia.

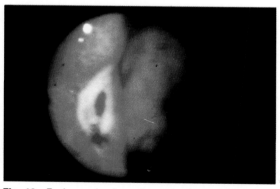

Fig. 46 Endoscopic view of gastric ulcer with a red dot indicating risk of re-haemorrhage.

15 | Coeliac Disease (Gluten Enteropathy) (1)

Definition

A sensitivity to gluten (which is found in wheat, barley and possibly oats) resulting in villous atrophy which responds to gluten withdrawal but is reproduced by re-challenge with gluten.

Epidemiology

Incidence is approximately one in 2500. It is familial in one patient in 10. It presents at any age in very diverse ways.

Pathology

Villous atrophy of jejunal mucosa with excess of intraepithelial lymphocytes.

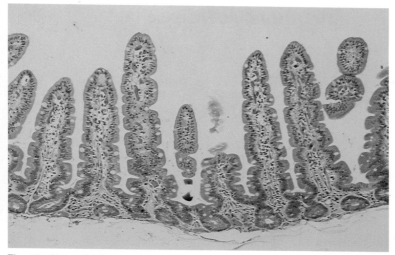

Fig. 47 Normal jejunum demonstrating tall villi.

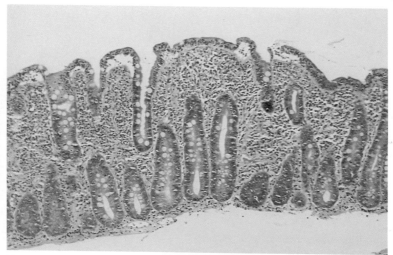

Fig. 48 Jejunum in coeliac disease showing sub-total villous atrophy and a marked inflammatory infiltrate.

15 | Coeliac Disease (2)

Presentation

General malaise, lethargy, abdominal discomfort and loose stools. Steatorrhoea is now found in a minority of patients. Features resulting from folate, iron and B_{12} deficiency may develop. Howell–Jolly bodies may be found in peripheral blood film due to concurrent hyposplenism (mechanism unknown). Deficiency of fat-soluble vitamins, particularly Vitamin D, may occur and patients may present with tetany. Less commonly short stature, delayed pubity, infertility and in severe cases finger clubbing occur.

Diagnosis

Clinical suspicion is important. Screen for hyposplenism and those deficiencies stated above. Antibodies to gluten or gliadin may be helpful. Diagnosis is confirmed or excluded by jejunal biopsy.

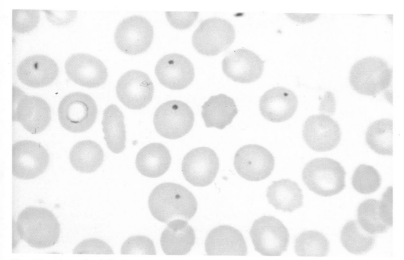

Fig. 49 Howell—Jolly bodies in coeliac disease.

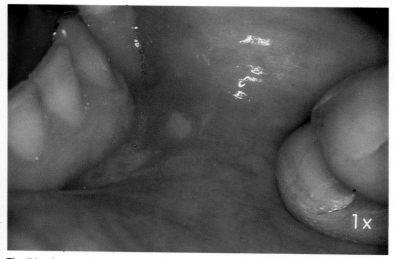

Fig. 50 Acute aphthous ulceration in the mouth sometimes associated with coeliac disease.

Treatment and progress

There is usually a dramatic response to gluten withdrawal. In the Longterm there is increased risk of malignancy, particularly of histiocytic lymphomas.

Comment

Other causes of villous atrophy include bacterial overgrowth, giardiasis, radiation, drugs and tropical sprue. Failure to respond to gluten withdrawal might indicate failure to adhere to diet or alternative diagnosis.

Associated features

These include dermatitis herpetiformis, a bullous rash usually seen over neck and elbows and nearly always associated with villous atrophy.

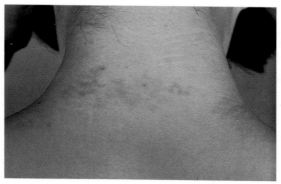

Fig. 51 Dermatitis herpetiformis complicating coeliac disease.

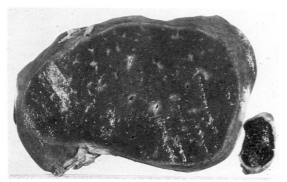

Fig. 52 Large liver and atrophic spleen in malignant lymphoma complicating coeliac disease.

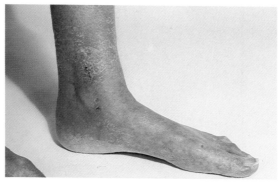

Fig. 53 Cryoglobulinaemia complicating coeliac disease.

16 | Malabsorption (1)

Definition

A syndrome occurring as a result of abnormal faecal excretion of fat (steatorrhoea) resulting from malabsorption of fats and soluble vitamins as well as carbohydrate and protein.

Pathogenesis

Causes can be classified into the following:
1. Primary mucosal abnormalities (coeliac disease, tropical sprue, disaccharidase deficiency).
2. Inadequate absorptive surfaces (gut resection, bypass or fistula).
3. Abnormalities of the intestinal wall, (Crohn's disease, infective enteritis, amyloidosis, drugs, e.g. cholestyramine or Neomycin, irradiation and eosinophylic gastroenteritis).
4. Lymphatic obstruction (lymphoma, tuberculosis or congenital lymphangiectasia).
5. Bacterial overgrowth (blind loop syndrome) and parasitic infections.
6. Chronic pancreatic insufficiency.
7. Exclusion or deficiency of conjugated bile salts.
8. Rare infection, including Whipple's disease and giardia lamblia.

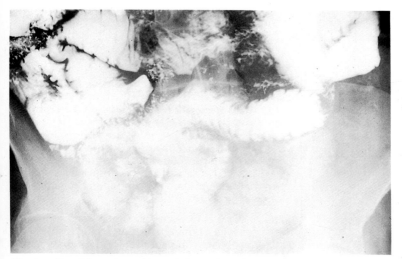

Fig. 54 Small bowel meal in malabsorption showing flocculation and dilatation of small intestine.

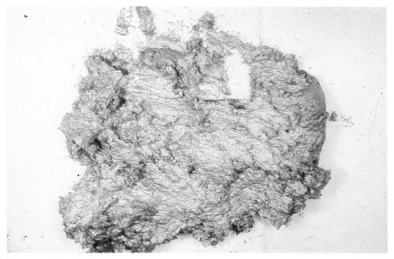

Fig. 55 Steatorrhoea.

16 | Malabsorption (2)

Symptoms

Steatorrhoea (pale, bulky, offensive and greasy stools which are difficult to flush away) is the classical presentation but this may be a relatively late feature. Earlier symptoms consist of vague abdominal discomfort or isolated nutritional deficiencies. These include anaemia (due to deficiency of iron, Vitamin B12 or folate), bone pain or tetany (deficiency of Vitamin D, calcium and magnesium) and spontaneous bruising (deficiency of Vitamin K).

Diagnosis

This is done in two stages. Firstly, to document the presence of malabsorption by illustrating increased faecal fat excretion or deficiency states (serum calcium, B_{12}, folate or iron). Secondly, to determine the cause; requiring in the first place jejunal biopsy and radiology of the small bowel. If both are normal, proceed to pancreatic function tests. The order of the tests performed will depend on clinical features.

Treatment

If possible correct the underlying cause. Symptomatically, a low-fat, high-protein diet may help. Correction of deficiency states is important.

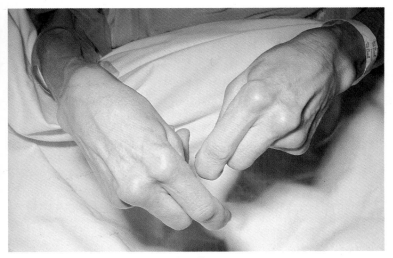

Fig. 56 Tetany complicating coeliac disease.

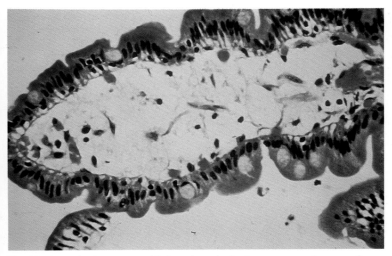

Fig. 57 Intestinal mucosa with lymphangiectasia, an unusual cause of malabsorption.

17 | Giardiasis

Definition

Infestation with *Giardia lamblia*.

Epidemiology

Worldwide distribution but particularly common in the Soviet Union. *Giardia lamblia* localised in the duodenum and upper jejunum.

Symptoms

Symptoms range from asymptomatic state to illness with acute or chronic diarrhoea. Rarely there is abdominal pain, nausea and vomiting. It may progress to frank malabsorption.

Diagnosis

It may be visualised in stool specimens but these may not always be present. Organisms can be seen on jejunal biopsy specimen.

Treatment

Metronidazole.

Comment

Empirical treatment with metronidazole is sometimes diagnostic if disease suspected. If disease is recurrent family contacts should also be treated. It may complicate an immunodeficiency state, particularly in IgA deficiency. A similar illness is caused by the organism *Balantidium* (Balantidiasis).

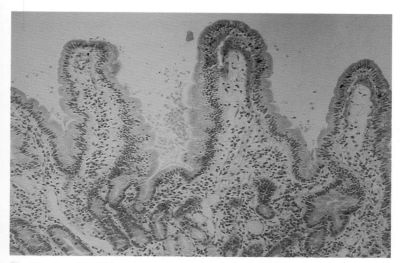

Fig. 58 Duodenal biopsy showing normal mucosa with adherent giardiasis.

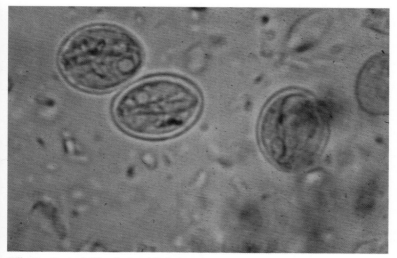

Fig. 59 Cyst of *Giardia lamblia* in stool.

18 | Uncommon Small Bowel Diseases (1)

Blind loop syndrome

This is caused by bacterial overgrowth in the small intestine. It may complicate almost any structural or motor abnormality of the small intestine. Most commonly it is seen in multiple jejunal diverticulosis, diabetes, Crohn's disease or following surgery, particularly when resulting in closed loop. It presents with symptoms of steatorrhoea and malabsorption, particularly of B_{12}. When disease is suspected empirical treatment with antibiotics (metronidazole or tetracycline) may result in diagnostic clinical improvement. Diagnosis is often difficult to confirm but C_{14} breath test and culture of jejunal aspirate may be helpful.

Whipple's Disease

A chronic disorder in which the small intestinal mucosa contains large numbers of abnormally foamy cells which stain positively with periodic acid Schiff (PAS) reagent. It presents with symptoms of malabsorption but also systemic features including lymphadenopathy, arthropathy and occasionally pericarditis or meningeal involvement. Diagnosis is normally confirmed histologically, usually by jejunal or lymph node biopsy. Prolonged treatment with tetracycline is curative and hence the condition is considered to be due to a presently undocumented infection.

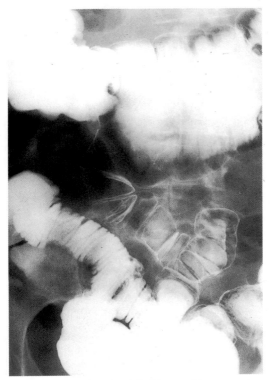

Fig. 60 X-ray showing blind loop with connection between stomach and transverse colon.

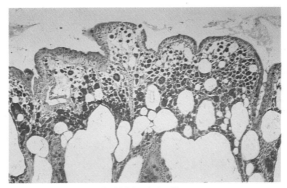

Fig. 61 Histology in Whipple's disease.

Uncommon Small Bowel Diseases (2)

Lymphangiectasia

A generalised disorder of the lymphatic system usually associated with the early onset of severe hypoproteinaemia. It is characterised by dilated telangiectatic lymphatic vessels in the mucosa of the small intestine which may be suspected radiologically and confirmed histologically by jejunal biopsy. Aetiology is unknown and treatment is empirical.

Eosinophilic gastroenteritis.

Characterised by infiltration of some part of the gastrointestinal tract with eosinophilic leucocytes. Clinical features include specific food intolerances, eosinophilia, diarrhoea and abdominal discomfort. Aetiology is unknown but most likely to be an allergy to an unknown antigen. Empirical treatment with corticosteroids may be effective. Dietary experimentation may find specific food intolerance which can then be omitted. It may be progressive and fatal.

Protein-losing enteropathy

Leakage of plasma proteins into the gastrointestinal tract resulting in hypoproteinaemia. It may complicate almost any GI disease, particularly Crohn's disease, gastric or colonic neoplasm and rarities such as Whipple's disease, menetrier's disease, eosinophilic gastroenteritis and lymphoma.

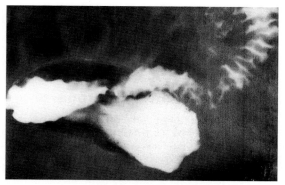

Fig. 62 Close up of small bowel in lymphangiectasia.

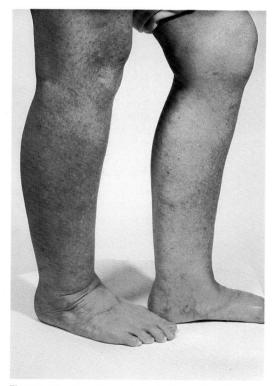

Fig. 63 Gross ankle oedema in hypoalbuminaemia secondary to lymphangiectasia.

Uncommom Small Bowel Diseases (3)

Short bowel syndrome

This is malabsorption following excision or bypass of the majority of the small intestine. It may occur following surgery for occlusion of the superior mesenteric artery or vein, or for extensive volvulus or internal strangulation. Treatment is initially with vigorous parenteral replacement therapy. Later there is transfer to complicated enteral feeding aimed at maximising absorption and minimising deficiency states. Occasionally, longterm parenteral alimentation is required.

Lymphoma

Any part of the bowel may be involved in disseminated lymphoma but primary gut lymphoma is rare. When it occurs it may complicate coeliac disease. The most common form seen in this situation is malignant histiocytosis of the intestine.

Vascular Diseases

The bowel may be involved in any vasculitic or arteritic process. It may present acutely with necrotic bowel or more obscurely with abdominal pain, fever or gastrointestinal haemorrhage. Diagnosis may require arteriography or biopsy. The most common form seen is abdominal pain complicated by Henoch—Schönlein's purpura.

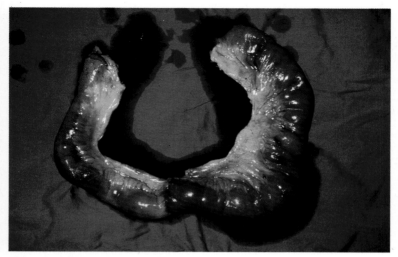

Fig. 64 Infarcted small bowel.

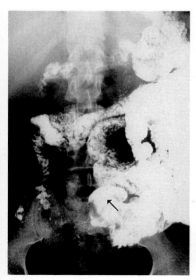

Fig. 65 Barium meal and follow through showing small intestinal lymphoma.

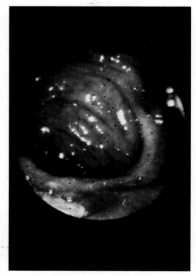

Fig. 66 Endoscopy of duodenum showing vasculitis.

Uncommon Small Bowel Diseases (4)

Systemic sclerosis

The oesophagus, small and large bowel may be involved. 80% of patients will have oesophageal involvement due to atrophy and replacement of the smooth muscle of the oesophagus by fibrous tissue. Small bowel involvement occurs in 60% and X-rays may show areas of thickening of the mucosa resulting in the 'stacked penny sign' or localised strictures. It may result in abdominal discomfort and malabsorption. Treatment of coexistent blind loop syndrome and nutritional deficiencies is important but in severe cases surgery may be required. It may be progressive and contribute to the patient's death.

Disaccharide intolerance

Lactose intolerance is relatively common and not usually associated with symptoms. When symptomatic, treatment with milk withdrawal may help. It usually presents with watery frothy stools and abdominal discomfort. Rarely, specific deficiencies of sucrase, glucoamylase or maltase may be demonstrated in the brush border on jejunal biopsy and specific dietary advice is then required.

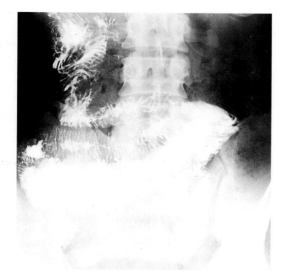

Fig. 67 Small bowel in scleroderma (stacked penny sign).

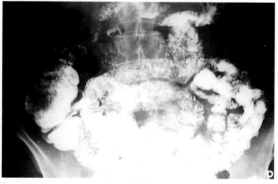

Fig. 68 Barium meal and follow-through showing changes in hypolactasia.

Uncommon small Bowel Diseases (5)

Ulcerative jejunitis

A rare condition in which multiple non-specific ulceration of the small intestine occurs. It presents with pain, malabsorption, perforation or haemorrhage. It is often a presenting feature of lymphoma.

Jejunal diverticulosis

An uncommon condition in which single or multiple diverticula are seen in the jejunum. These are more common with advancing age. They may be asymptomatic or complicated by bacterial overgrowth syndrome with diarrhoea, B_{12} deficiency, perforation or bleeding.

Surgical treatment is only rarely required.

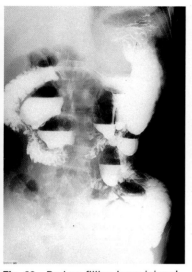

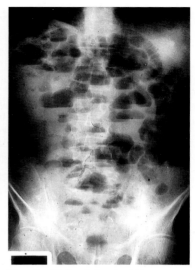

Fig. 69 Barium filling large jejunal diverticular disease.

Fig. 70 Plain abdominal X-ray showing fluid levels in multiple jejunal diverticulae.

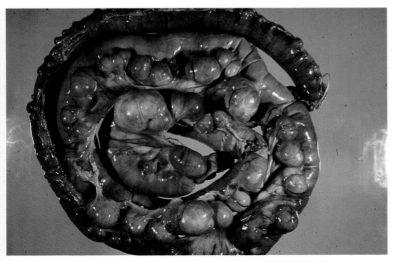

Fig. 71 Pathological specimen of small bowel showing multiple diverticulae.

19 | Carcinoid Syndrome

Definition

A rare syndrome resulting from abnormal production of 5-hydroxytryptophan and other substances, such as histamine and prostaglandins. These are produced from tumours derived from the APUD cells most commonly found in the small bowel but also from the stomach, rectum and elsewhere.

Symptoms

These only occur once extensive liver metastasis has occurred. Symptoms include diarrhoea, abdominal cramps and episodic flushing, leading to telangiectasia and occasionally pellagra-like skin rashes, bronchospasm or valvular heart lesions.

Diagnosis

Clinical suspicion is important. Measurement of 24-hour urine 5HIAA is usually diagnostic. In difficult cases it can be confirmed by liver biopsy.

Treatment

The condition has a long natural history and treatment with serotonin antagonists (methysergide), antihistamine or methyldopa may give symptomatic relief. Chemotherapy, embolisation or surgery may be required.

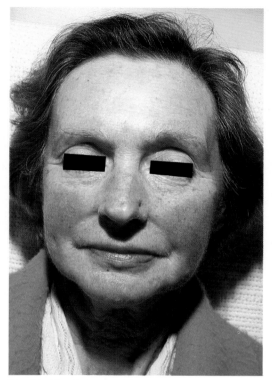

Fig. 72 The facial flush in carcinoid syndrome.

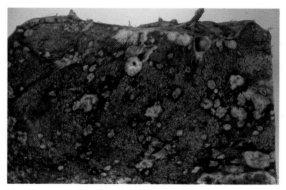

Fig. 73 Liver involvement with carcinoid.

20 | Amyloidosis

Definition

Deposition in any tissues of an amorphous substance. There are two types:
1. Primary with deposition of an immunoglobulin, a variant of myeloma.
2. Secondary deposition of abnormal protein following longstanding inflammatory conditions.

Symptoms

These can be various depending on which organ is most involved.

Diagnosis

Amyloid can be seen on rectal biopsies in 70% of cases, particularly if stained with congo red. It can also be seen in other tissues including liver and small intestine.

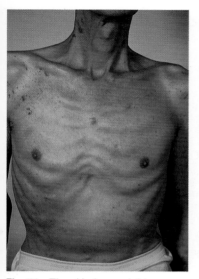

Fig. 74 The skin in amyloid.

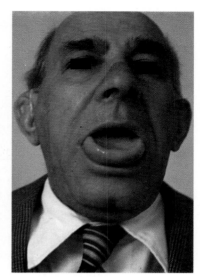

Fig. 75 Large tongue in amyloid.

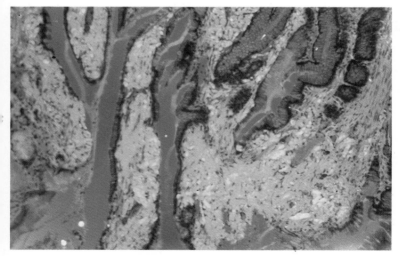

Fig. 76 Amyloidosis in intestinal mucosa.

21 | Inflammatory Bowel Disease (1)

Definition

A chronic non-specific inflammatory condition of the intestine. There are two main types: ulcerative colitis which affects only the colon starting distally, and Crohn's disease which may involve any part of the GI tract, particularly the small intestine. The term proctitis describes patients in whom the disease is confined to the rectum. Many patients with inflammatory bowel disease (IBD) cannot be accurately classified into either group.

Epidemiology

Approximately 1 in 1000. More common in females. Any age but biggest peak at 20–30 years. Familial tendency and more common in Jews. Aetiology is unknown, but possibly an infective agent or other antigen is involved. The incidence of Crohn's disease, particularly the colonic form, is increasing.

Pathology

In ulcerative colitis superficial diffuse inflammatory infiltrate with or without ulceration. Later pseudopolyps can form. In Crohn's disease focal full-thickness inflammatory infiltrate with fissures. Granulomas present in about 50% of cases. Normal areas may separate diseased areas (skip lesions).

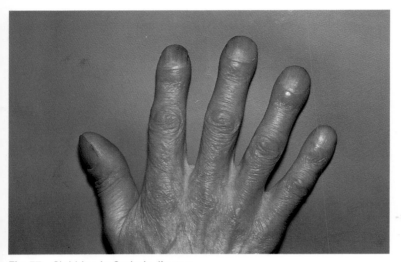

Fig. 77 Clubbing in Crohn's disease.

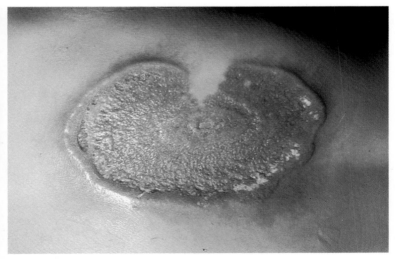

Fig. 78 Close-up of pyoderma gangrenosum.

21 | Inflammatory Bowel Disease (2)

Complications

Note
Some complications are more common in ulcerative colitis , others in Crohn's disease (see pages 65 and 67).

Gastro-intestinal
Perforation, haemorrhage, stricture formation, toxic megacolon, fistulas and fissures.

Skin
Erythema nodosum, pyoderma gangrenosum.

Musculo-skeletal
Arthralgia, large joint sero-negative arthritis, ankylosing spondylitis, sacroileitis.

Liver
Fatty change, pericholangitis, sclerosing cholangitis, chronic active hepatitis, gallstones, bile duct carcinoma and granulomatous hepatitis.

General
Finger clubbing, mouth ulcers, iritis, uveitis, amyloid, oxylate kidney stones.

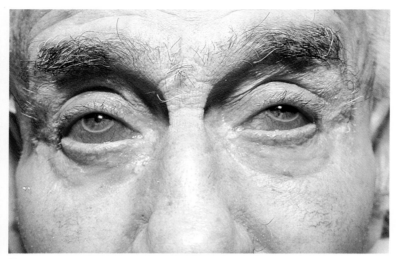

Fig. 79 Uveitis associated with IBD.

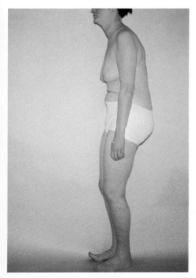

Fig. 80 Posture in ankylosing spondylitis associated with IBD.

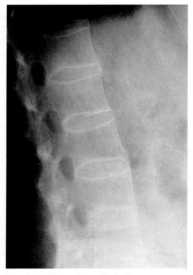

Fig. 81 X-ray in ankylosing spondylitis.

Inflammatory Bowel Disease (3)

Ulcerative colitis

Presentation

It usually presents with diarrhoea containing blood and mucus. It may present with systemic illness or complications.

X-ray findings

Barium enema shows mucosal irregularity, ulceration, loss of haustral pattern, shortening of colon, pseudopolyps or benign stricture. Backwash ileitis occurs but there is no true small bowel involvement.

Sigmoidoscopy

Diffuse inflammation with loss of vascular pattern, friable or haemorrhagic mucosa. Sometimes pseudopolyps form.

Specific complications

1. Increased risk of colonic cancer— approximately 1% risk per year in patients with total colitis.
2. Sclerosing cholangitis.
3. Bile duct carcinoma.
4. Toxic megacolon which requires urgent hospitalisation and early surgery if it fails to settle.

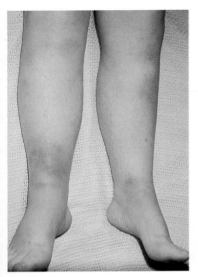

Fig. 82 Erythema nodosum of the legs.

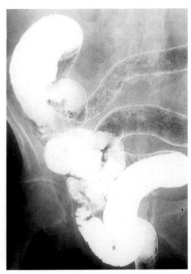

Fig. 83 Barium enema showing featureless colon in longstanding ulcerative colitis.

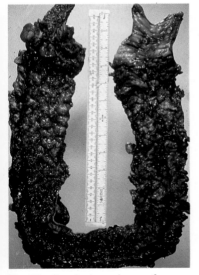

Fig. 84 Surgical specimen of longstanding ulcerative colitis.

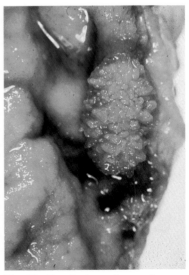

Fig. 85 Surgical specimen of dysplasia complicating ulcerative colitis.

Inflammatory Bowel Disease (4)

Crohn's disease of the small bowel

Presentation

Presentation can be very varied with abdominal pain or mass, weight loss, general malaise, anaemia and diarrhoea being the most prominent. It can present with complications when underlying disease may be relatively occult.

X-ray findings

A barium meal and follow-through shows mucosal irregularities, segmental narrowing and stricture formation. Skip lesions and the string sign often with gross distortion of the small intestine can be seen.

Diagnosis

Colonoscopy may give useful information and enable biopsies of the colon or terminal ileum but sometimes laparotomy is required to confirm diagnosis.

Special complications

1. Fistula formation.
2. Malabsorption.
3. Gallstones.
4. Amyloid.
5. Granulomatous hepatitis.
6. Oxalate kidney stones.
7. Small intestinal adenocarcinomas.

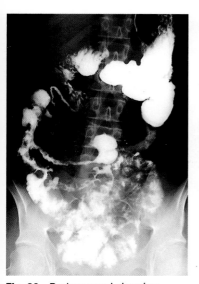

Fig. 86 Barium meal showing segments of Crohn's disease.

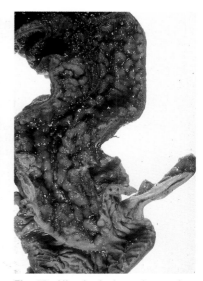

Fig. 87 Histological specimen of Crohn's disease showing full thickness changes.

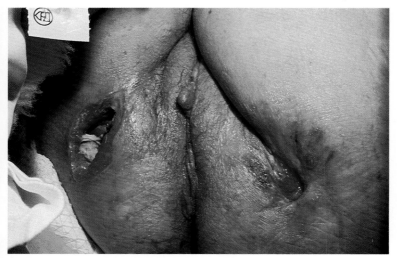

Fig. 88 Ano-rectal fistulas in Crohn's disease.

Crohn's colitis

Presentation

Bloody diarrhoea with mucus. Abdominal pain and complications are more common than in ulcerative colitis. There may be coexistent small bowel disease.

X-ray findings

A barium enema may show discrete aphthous ulceration. These may become linear ulcers and there may be cobblestoning, pseudopolyp formation and fissures leading to sinus, fistula or abscess formation. The disease is often segmental.

Colonoscopy

Discrete ulceration with apparently normal mucosa between. Sometimes frank cobblestoning of the mucosa with severe ulceration.

Special complications

Perianal disease is very common (fissures, fistula, abscesses).

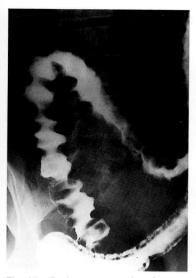

Fig. 89 Barium enema showing Crohn's disease with deep ulcers.

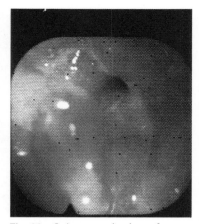

Fig. 90 Colonoscopic view of Crohn's disease with ulceration.

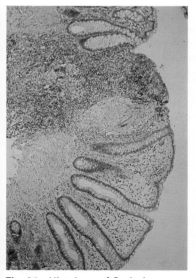

Fig. 91 Histology of Crohn's granuloma.

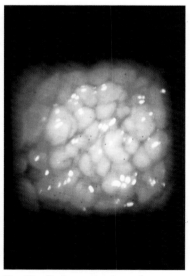

Fig. 92 Endoscopic view of cobblestoning in stomach due to Crohn's disease.

Inflammatory Bowel Disease (6)

Treatment

General

General measures and support. Sensible nutritional advice. Codeine phosphate or Imodium may help to control diarrhoea.

Specific

Salazopyrin or Asacol (continuous). Topical steroids or systemic steroids are used when there is no response to the above measures. Intravenous steroids may be required in severe cases.

Other

Azathioprine or 5-mercaptopurine, metronidazole, particularly for anal complications in Crohn's disease. Exclusion diet may help. Surgery for complications, e.g. haemorrhage, perforation, fistula or toxic megacolon. Also when medical treatment has failed, particularly when excess of steroid dosage is required. In ulcerative colitis total colectomy with ileostomy or some form of ileorectal anastomosis is curative. In Crohn's disease local excision should be performed when possible.

Comment

Most patients with Crohn's disease will require surgery at some time but this is not curative. The disease is likely to recur although sometimes after prolonged remission.

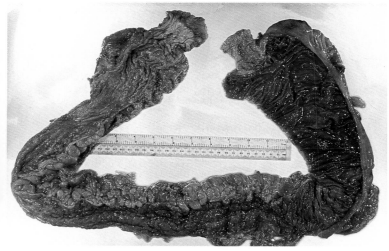

Fig. 93 Surgical specimen of Crohn's disease.

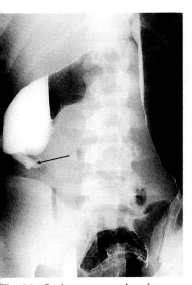

Fig. 94 Barium enema showing carcinoma complicating longstanding ulcerative colitis.

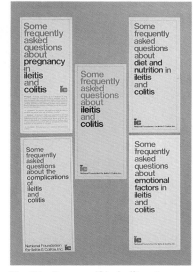

Fig. 95 Some self-help literature useful in the treatment of patients with inflammatory bowel disease.

Infectious Diarrhoea

All the following should be considered and excluded in the differential diagnosis of idiopathic inflammatory bowel disease.

Campylobacter enterocolitis

Perhaps the most common cause of infectious diarrhoea in the UK. Presents with fever or bloody diarrhoea. May also develop acute abdomen or reactive arthropathy. Responds to Erythromycin.

Salmonella/Shigella

Presents with acute dysentery occasionally complicated by major complication of bleeding or perforation. Usually settles spontaneously except in the case of *Salmonella typhi* (typhoid fever) when antibiotics are mandatory (ampicillin or chloramphenicol).

Amoebiasis

This should be considered in patients recently returning from overseas travel. It may present with diarrhoea or with involvement with other organs particularly liver abscesses. Usually responds to metronidazole.

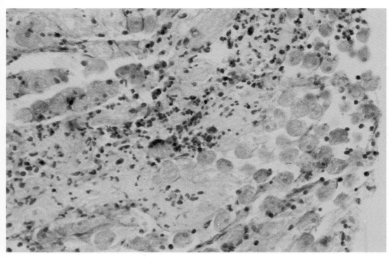

Fig. 96 Histology of amoebic dysentery showing amoebae.

23 | Irritable Bowel Syndrome

Definition

Motility disorder primarily affecting large bowel but involving the whole of the GI tract.

Epidemiology

Very common, affecting up to one-third of the population in some form. Affects any age and is a disease of Western civilisation, possibly due to reduced fibre intake. Psychic factors are also important.

Symptoms

Pain related to bowel movements, diarrhoea or constipation with the passage of mucus. These may be severe and varied and it is now recognised that upper GI symptoms, such as anorexia, nausea and dyspepsia, can result from a similar problem affecting the upper GI tract.

Diagnosis

It is important to exclude other diseases which may mimic this syndrome, particularly neoplastic disease or inflammatory bowel disease. Sigmoidoscopy with biopsy, barium enema or colonoscopy may therefore be required, particularly in elderly patients.

Treatment

Reassurance, dietary advice regarding increased fibre intake and the intermittent use of bulking agents. Antispasmodic or antidepressants may be useful.

Date	Time	Amount	Colour	Consistency	FOB
6-9-87	0.8-15	65 gms	brown	pellets + mucus	-ve
"	10-0.5	30 gms	brown	hard	-ve
"	13-20	45 gms	brown	firm	-ve
"	18-45	60 gms	brown	pellets	-ve
7-9-87	08-10	80 gms	brown	hard	neg.
"	09-50	35 gms	brown	hard + mucus	-ve
8-9-87	08-20	90 gms	brown	pellets	neg.
"	10-00	45 gms	brown	firm	-ve
"	12-35	40 gms	brown	hard	-ve
"	14-45	30 gms	brown	firm	-ve

Fig. 97 A typical stool chart in the irritable bowel syndrome with frequent small stools, normal total daily stool weight and nocturnal sparing.

24 | Diverticular Disease

Definition

Acquired herniation of mucosa and submucosa through muscle wall of the colon. The term diverticular disease encompasses diverticulosis, the presence of uninflamed diverticula and diverticulitis when these become inflamed.

Epidemiology

Incidence increases with age and one-third of patients over 60 years are estimated to be affected. Incidence is particularly high in Western civilisation due to dietary changes, particularly reduced fibre intake, which results in increased colonic pressure.

Symptoms

Usually asymptomatic but may present with acute or chronic haemorrhage, or with evidence of inflammation with pain, altering bowel habit, and a tender mass.

Treatment

Patients with asymptomatic disease should be recommended a high fibre diet. Bulking agents and antispasmodics may help control symptoms. Acute episodes of inflammation can be treated with antibiotics but surgery may be needed for this or for complications which include fistula, obstruction, abscess formation or peritonitis. Colonoscopy is often needed to exclude the presence of a coexistent polyp.

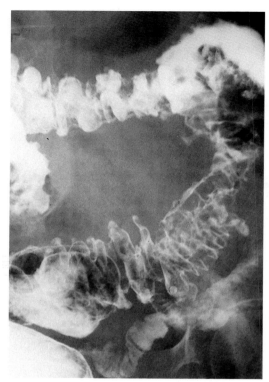

Fig. 98 Barium enema showing severe sigmoid diverticular disease.

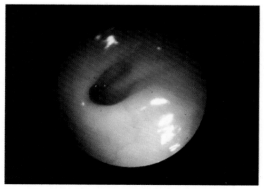

Fig. 99 Colonoscopic view of mouth of sigmoid diverticulum.

| # Colonic and Rectal Carcinoma (1)

Definition

Adenocarcinoma originating from colonic mucosa. 70% are found in the rectum or recto-sigmoid area.

Epidemiology

Incidence is increasing in Western civilisation probably due to some dietary change, possibly a decrease in the amount of fibre eaten. Abnormal bile salts, altered colonic bacteria and familial factors may be involved. There is increased incidence in patients with villous adenomas, ulcerative colitis and familial polyposis, and in Gardner's syndrome.

Symptoms

Change of bowel habit with alternating diarrhoea and constipation, sometimes with blood or mucus is most common presentation. May present with metastatic disease, e.g. with weight loss or as a surgical emergency with obstruction or perforation. Rectal examination, sigmoidoscopy and barium enema or colonoscopy usually confirm the diagnosis.

Treatment

Surgical, although chemotherapy as adjuvant therapy has a small beneficial effect. Prognosis depends on the extent of disease.

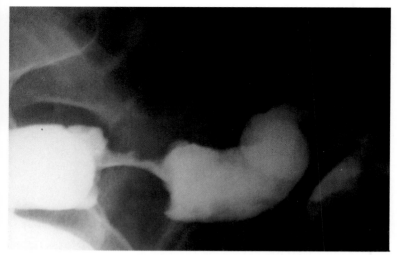

Fig. 100 Barium enema showing rectal carcinoma ('apple core lesion').

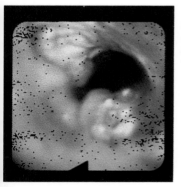

Fig. 101 Colonoscopy showing colonic cancer.

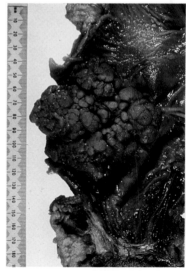

Fig. 102 Histological specimen of villus adenoma.

Comment

In many cases this is thought to originate as adenomatous polyps which slowly grow and then become malignant. Early diagnosis by screening for occult blood loss and endoscopic removal of these polyps at an early stage may therefore offer hope of disease prevention and early diagnosis of cancer.

Colonic polyps

Definition

It may be hyperplastic, adenomatous or villous.

Symptoms

Altered bowel habits, lower GI blood loss and the passage of mucus should suggest diagnosis. Villous adenomas may present with hypokalaemia due to potassium loss. It may be a chance finding in patients being investigated for other reasons.

Treatment

Hyperplastic polyps are benign but adenomatous or villous ones should be removed in view of the cancer risk. This can be achieved endoscopically in most cases but occasionally surgical resection is required. Polyps may re-form and patients need to be kept under regular review.

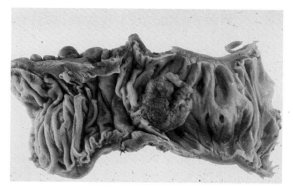

Fig. 103 Surgical specimen of carcinoma of the colon.

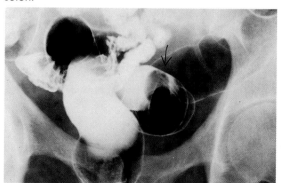

Fig. 104 Barium enema showing polyp.

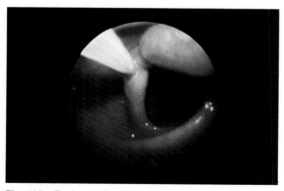

Fig. 105 Endoscopic view of polyp about to be removed by snare.

Hereditary Polyposis Syndrome (1)

Familial polyposis

An autosomal dominant condition with multiple adenomas in the colon. The significance of the condition is that 95% of patients will develop adenocarcinomas and thus prophylactic colectomy is indicated.

Gardner's syndrome

A dominantly inherited syndrome of adenomatous polyposis of the colon, rectum and occasionally stomach and small intestine. It is associated with osteomas, soft tissue abnormality including epidermoid cysts, fibromas and lipomas, and supernumerary teeth. Risk of malignancy is similar to familial polyposis.

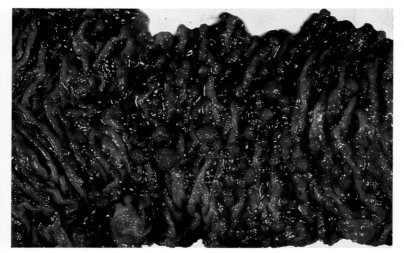

Fig. 106 Surgical specimen of multiple familial polyposis.

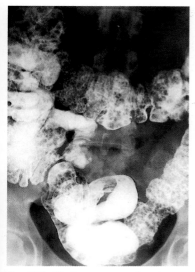

Fig. 107 Barium enema showing familial polyposis of colon.

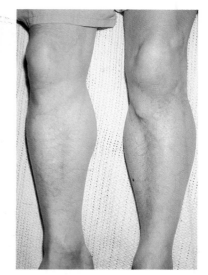

Fig. 108 Exostosis in Gardner's syndrome associated with colonic polyp.

| # Hereditary Polyposis Syndrome (2)

Peutz—Jeghers syndrome

Dominantly inherited condition with hamartomas in the gastrointestinal tract associated in all but a few cases with melanotic pigmentation of the lips and buccal mucosa. It can be complicated by haemorrhage or intussusception but the risk of malignancy is low.

Cronkhite—Canada syndrome

Very rare. There are pseudopolyps in the intestinal tract from the stomach to the rectum which result from mucinous cyst dilatation. Associated features are alopecia, oncodystrophy, pigmentation, malabsorption and protein-losing enteropathy. This is not an inherited condition.

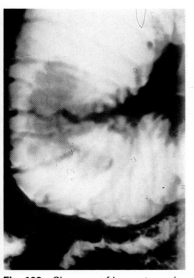

Fig. 109 Close-up of hamartoma in the small intestine of a patient with Peutz-Jeghers syndrome (see also Fig. 44).

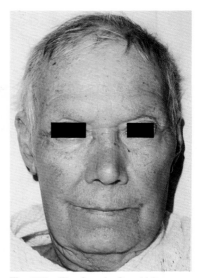

Fig. 110 The face in Cronkhite–Canada syndrome.

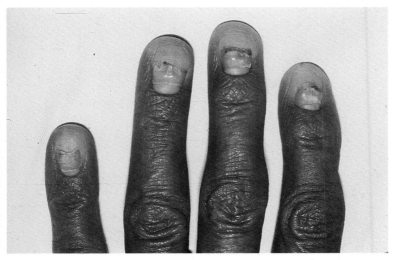

Fig. 111 Pigmentation and loss of fingernails in Cronkhite–Canada syndrome.

Definition

Acute diarrhoeal illness following antibiotic therapy caused by bacterially produced toxins.

Aetiology

This is most commonly seen after treatment with clindamycin but it may complicate the use of any antibiotic. Toxins produced by *Clostridium difficile* are the most common cause, although other toxins probably produce similar illness. This toxin can be detected in the laboratory.

Symptoms

Oral vancomycin or metronidazole. If toxic megacolon occurs colectomy may be required.

Comment

C. difficile is occasionally found in normal colons and it is assumed that the use of antibiotics allows rapid overgrowth.

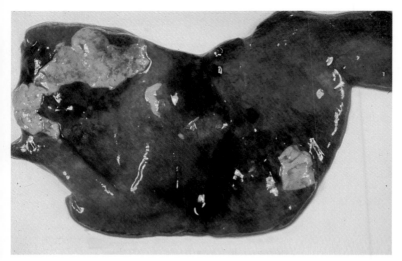

Fig. 112 Surgical specimen showing pseudomembrane in antibiotic-associated colitis.

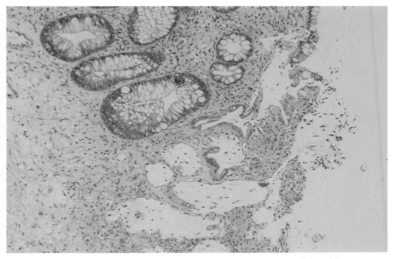

Fig. 113 Histological specimen of pseudomembranous colitis with a pronounced inflammatory exudate.

Ischaemic Colitis

Definition

Colitis due to interruption of arterial blood supply.

Epidemiology

This usually occurs in the elderly, especially those with cardiovascular disease. It may complicate atrial fibrillation (due to embolisation). Any part of the colon can be affected but the splenic flexure is the site most commonly involved.

Symptoms

Initially there is abdominal pain and diarrhoea with the passage of blood longterm. It may progress to stricture formaton. It often settles on symptomatic treatment, although surgery is sometimes required.

Diagnosis

Clinical suspicion is important. Endoscopic appearance, biopsy or barium studies are usually confirmatory.

Radiation colitis

Definition

The large and small bowel are sensitive to large doses of radiotherapy and this may result in severe diarrhoea.

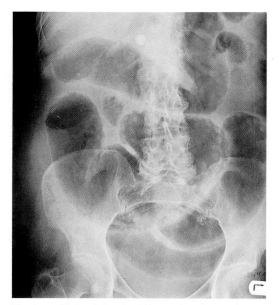

Fig. 114 Plain abdominal X-ray showing toxic megacolon with finger printing due to ischaemic colitis.

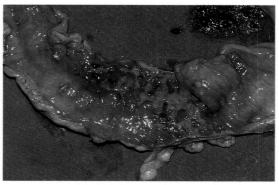

Fig. 115 Surgical specimen of ischaemic colitis.

29 | Angiodysplasia

Definition

Arterial–venous abnormality in the colonic mucosa usually on the right side. It is probably acquired rather than inherited.

Symptoms

It is often asymptomatic but may present with recurrent lower GI blood loss.

Diagnosis

It may be seen as a cherry-red spot at colonoscopy but arteriography may be required for confirmation.

Treatment

It can be diathermied at colonoscopy but may require surgical excision if bleeding continues. Fatal haemorrhage rarely occurs. Diagnosis should be considered in patients with iron deficiency anaemia in whom no cause for blood loss can be found.

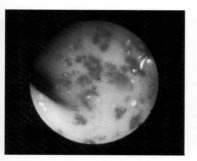

Fig. 116 Endoscopic view of angiodysplasia of the colon.

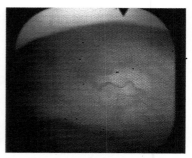

Fig. 117 Further endoscopic view of angiodysplasia of the colon.

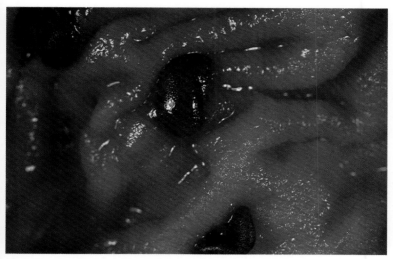

Fig. 118 Surgical specimen of vascular lesion of the colon.

Hirschsprung's disease

Caused by a congenital lack of ganglion cells in the intramural plexus of the large bowel. The affected segment may be very short. Presents at a young age with severe constipation. Barium enema may reveal narrowed segment with dilated colon proximally. Rectal biopsy may confirm diagnosis if submucosal tissue is included. Symptomatic treatment may be helpful but most patients require surgery.

Megacolon

Hugely dilated colon associated with constipation. Most commonly it is idiopathic or psychogenic but it may result from laxative abuse, neurological disorders and a number of other conditions.

Melanosis coli

Abnormally brown and pigmented colonic mucosa thought to result from longterm purgative abuse. It is asymptomatic but indicates laxative abuse.

Tuberculosis

TB can affect the bowel and be confused with GI malignancy.

Laxative abuse

A syndrome of diarrhoea often associated with weight loss due to secretive intake of excessive purgatives. It indicates severe psychological problems.

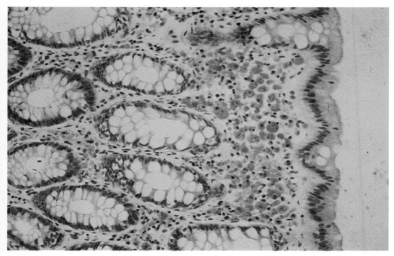

Fig. 119 Histology of melanosis coli showing brown pigment.

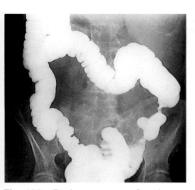

Fig. 120 Barium enema of patient proved later to have tuberculosis (see Fig. 121).

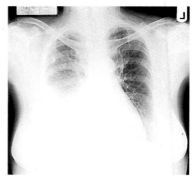

Fig. 121 Chest X-ray of same patient.

Endometriosis

This may sometimes involve the colon resulting in pain, diarrhoea and other symptoms.

Solitary ulcer syndrome

Benign ulceration of the rectum considered to be due to prolapse of the mucosa or to self-digitation. Symptoms include diarrhoea, discomfort and mucus PR. Diagnosis is confirmed on sigmoidoscopy and rectal biopsy. More than one ulcer may be present. Often mistakenly diagnosed as inflammatory bowel disease or neoplasm.

Colitis cystica profunda

Benign mucus-filled polypoid lesions in the colon. Diagnosis may be confirmed by sigmoidoscopy and biopsy. No specific treatment is necessary as the condition is benign.

Pneumotosis cystoides intestinalis

Gas-filled cysts in the rectum and colon which may be mistaken for multiple polyposis. Gas can be seen on plain abdominal film and the diagnosis confirmed by biopsies. The disease is occasionally associated with chronic lung disease. Treatment, when necessary, is with hyperbaric oxygen.

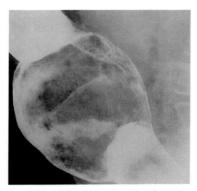

Fig. 122 A barium showing faecal impaction in Hirschsprung's disease.

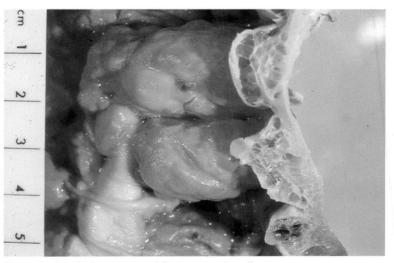

Fig. 123 Surgical specimen of *Pneumocystis coli*.

Anal–Rectal Disease

Haemorrhoids

Dilated veins of the haemorrhoidal plexus. A very common condition (50% of patients over 50 years). May be internal or external. Classified as first-degree if in the anal canal, second-degree if there is prolapse on defecation but it reduces spontaneously, third-degree if it requires manual reduction, and fourth-degree if it is irreducible. It presents with haemorrhage (bright red blood on toilet paper), prolapse, mucus discharge or itching. It may become thrombosed when extremely painful. Treatment is aimed at softening the stool, but it may require injection, rubber band ligation or surgery.

Fissure-in-ano

A split in the anal mucosa usually resulting from straining. 90% are posterior. It presents with pain on defecation or haemorrhage. It may heal spontaneously if stool softeners are used but it may require dilatation using special anal dilators.

Pruritus ani

Itching in the perianal region which may result from (1) anal-rectal diseases, (2) dermatological conditions, (3) infection, (4) parasites, (5) poor hygiene, (6) psychogenic causes. Treatment is unsatisfactory but hygiene is most important. Hydrocortisone cream may be helpful.

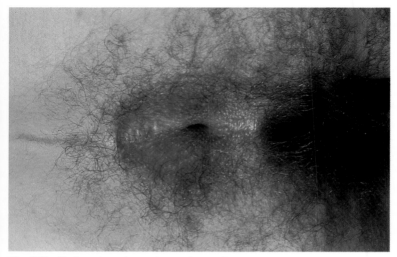

Fig. 124 Peri-anal erythema in pruritus ani.

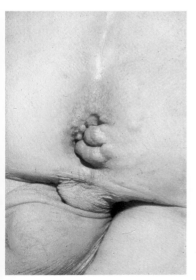

Fig. 125 Haemorrhoids.

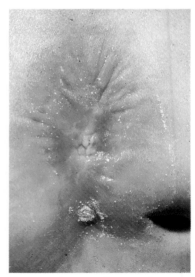

Fig. 126 Crohn's disease of anus.

32 | Intestinal Parasites

Ascariasis (Round worm)
Ova are spread by faecal—oral contact. They hatch in the small intestine, penetrate the intestinal wall, enter the circulation and return to the small bowel by migrating through the pulmonary alveoli. Symptoms are haemoptysis, eosinophilia and pulmonary inflammation (Loeffler's syndrome). Abdominal symptoms include intestinal obstruction.

Ankylostomiasis (Hook worm)
Similar life-cycle to ascariasis. Abdominal symptoms include diarrhoea and iron deficiency anaemia.

Oxyuriasis (Thread worm)
Adult worms live in the right colon but females migrate to the rectum to deposit eggs resulting in pruritus ani.

Strongyloidiasis
Similar life-cycle to Ascaris. Skin irritation during skin penetration and lung symptoms during transalveolar migration. Diarrhoea and malabsorption may occur.

Taeniasis (Tape worm)
Encysted cercariae are eaten in undercooked pork (*Taenia solium*) or beef (*T. sageneta*). Requires an intermediate host. Symptoms include abdominal pain and weight loss.

Trichinosis
It results from eating measly pork (containing cysts of *Trichinella spiralis*) and presents with abdominal pain, vomiting and diarrhoea, and generalised allergic manifestation.

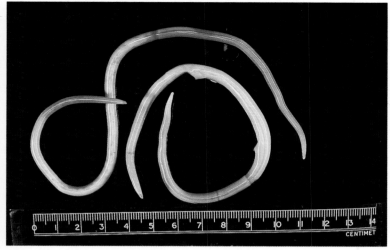

Fig. 127 Ascaris or roundworm.

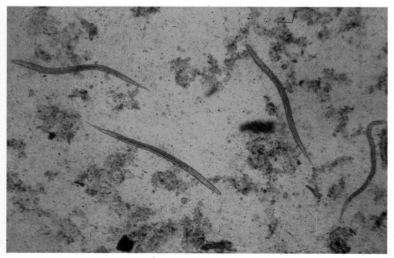

Fig. 128 *Strongyloides stercoralis.*

Miscellaneous Conditions

Appendicitis

Acute inflammation of the appendix—
sometimes caused by a faecolith. It presents
with central abdominal pain which shifts over
several hours to the right iliac fossa. Fever,
vomiting and peritonism commonly present. It is
important to differentiate other causes of such
symptoms particularly Crohn's disease or
mesenteric abnormalities. Laparotomy may be
necessary to confirm the diagnosis and
treatment is by surgical excision. If treatment is
delayed the complications include peritonitis due
to perforation or abscess formation. It is doubtful
whether chronic appendicitis exists and it is risky
to attribute longstanding symptoms to this
diagnosis.

Meckel's diverticulum

This is the most frequent congenital abnormality
of the intestinal tract occurring in about 2% of
patients. It is usually asymptomatic but it may
present with haemorrhage or pain due to
ulceration of ectopic gastric epithelium.

Intestinal angina

A rare syndrome due to extensive atheroma of
the intestinal arteries. It presents with severe
pain following meals, weight loss and diarrhoea.
Although a bruit may be audible the diagnosis is
difficult and may require arteriography for
confirmation. Surgical treatment is occasionally
successful.

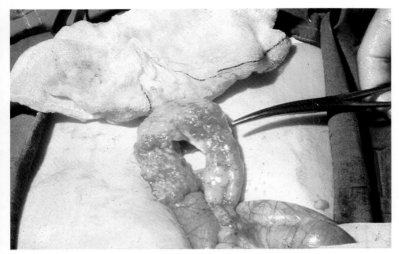

Fig. 129 Surgical specimen of inflamed appendix.

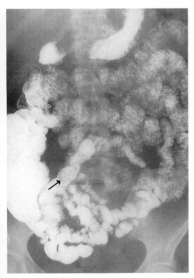

Fig. 130 Meckel's diverticulum showing on barium meal and follow through.

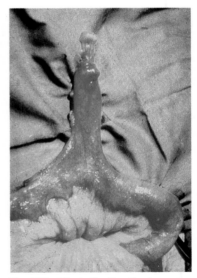

Fig. 131 Meckel's diverticulum at laparotomy.

34 | **Acute Pancreatitis**

Definition

Acute inflammation of the pancreas which can be haemorrhagic. It is particularly common in alcoholics and can be caused by cholelithiasis and a number of different drugs.

Symptoms

Severe pain and peritonism, nausea and vomiting, fever and shock. It may be complicated by ileus, coagulation abnormalities, and pseudocyst formation. Rarely there is GI haemorrhage, pleural effusions, subcutaneous fat necrosis, hypocalcaemia and colonic stricture. There may be signs of retroperitoneal haemorrhage (Grey Turner's sign).

Diagnosis and treatment

Usually confirmed by demonstration of high serum amylase. Treatment is symptomatic with pain relief and care of fluid balance. Enzyme inhibitors, such as Trasicor, are of unproven value. It is important to distinguish acute pancreatitis from other causes of an acute abdomen, particularly perforation, as these can also result in an elevated serum amylase. Mortality apporaches 50% and may progress to chronic pancreatitis.

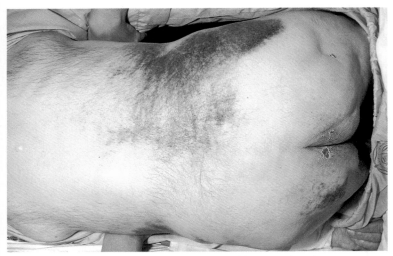

Fig. 132 Grey Turner's sign in acute pancreatitis, posterior view.

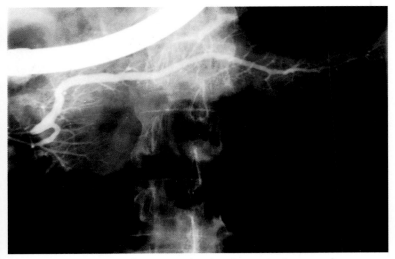

Fig. 133 Endoscopic pancreatography showing early changes of pancreatitis with beading of the duct.

35 | Chronic Pancreatitis

Definition

Chronic inflammation of the pancreas which may become calcified. Common in alcoholics and may be caused by cholelithiasis, hyperparathyroidism or following trauma.

Symptoms

Abdominal pain, often described as a dull boring ache, sometimes radiating through to the back. Pain sometimes relieved by assuming squatting position. Systemic symptoms such as weight loss, malabsorption, diabetes and depression are common.

Diagnosis and treatment

Serum amylase may be slightly elevated. Plain abdominal film may show pancreatic calcification. The gland can be outlined by ultrasound and CAT scanning and the pancreatic duct can be outlined at ERCP. Exocrine function can be assessed by the non-invasive PABA test or by Lundh meal. Pain relief and moral support are important. Local nerve blocks or major surgery may be required in difficult cases either to correct a ductal stenosis or for symptomatic relief.

Comment

A very difficult condition to treat as patients are frequently alcohol-dependent. It is often difficult to distinguish it from carcinoma of the pancreas.

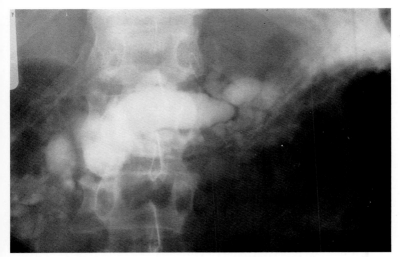

Fig. 134 Endoscopic pancreatogram showing hugely dilated pancreatic duct in chronic pancreatitis.

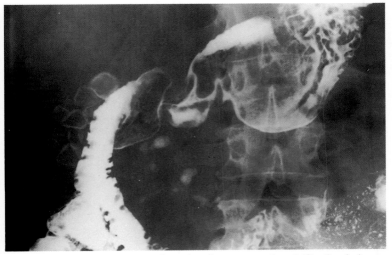

Fig. 135 Barium meal on a patient showing pancreatic calcification in large pancreatic loop and opaque gall stone.

36 | Carcinoma of the Pancreas

Definition

Adenocarcinoma arising from pancreas. 70% occur in the head of the pancreas. It is more common in males and has increasing incidence. Predisposing factors include smoking, heavy alcohol intake and possibly diabetes and coffee drinking.

Symptoms

Symptoms are often vague and ill-defined. Pain, indistinguishable from that of chronic pancreatitis, may be present. Systemic symptoms are weight loss, depression and diabetes especially, and rarely GI haemorrhage, thrombophlebitis and subcutaneous fat necrosis. Most patients eventually become jaundiced due to bile duct obstruction and this is a common presentation.

Diagnosis

It can be difficult to distinguish from chronic pancreatitis. Needle biopsy under ultrasound control may prevent unnecessary laparotomy but surgery is often required to confirm diagnosis. A barium meal may show infiltration into the duodenum. It can be difficult to distinguish it from carcinoma of the ampulla of Vater. Surgery is usually palliative and attempts at excision are very rarely curative.

Comment

One year survival is less than 10% and the disease is a very difficult one to treat.

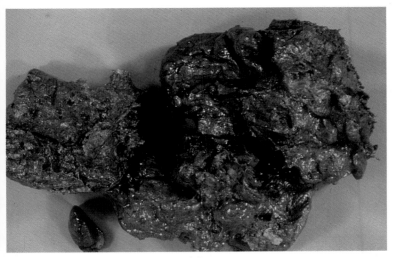

Fig. 136 Silver stool in carcinoma of the pancreas.

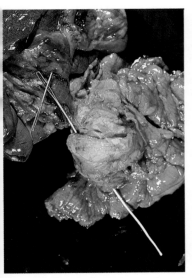

Fig. 137 Surgical specimen of carcinoma of head of the pancreas.

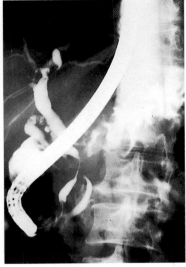

Fig. 138 ERCP showing stricture of pancreatic and bile ducts in carcinoma of the pancreas.

37 | **The Liver**

Function

The function of the liver is diverse and as well as bilirubin metabolism includes protein synthesis and degradation, storage and release of fats and carbohydrate, and detoxification of drugs and toxins. An important role is hormone metabolism. It also has immunological functions.

Jaundice—classification

Jaundice can be classified as prehepatic, hepatocellular or posthepatic. The distinction between types is not always clearcut.

Prehepatic
This occurs in haemolytic anaemias (familial, immunological or drug-induced). There is splenomegaly, reticulocytosis and anaemia in severe cases. Urobilinogen will be found in urine and haptoglobins may be absent in the serum. It is also seen in congenital hyperbilirubinaemias, most commonly Gilbert's syndrome.

Hepatocellular
Parenchymal liver disease is either acute or chronic. Predominant biochemical abnormality is an increase in transaminase but occasionally intrahepatic cholestasis may be prominent.

Posthepatic
This is due to obstruction of bile ducts which in turn is usually due to cancer or gallstones. The predominant abnormality is an increase in alkaline phosphatase.

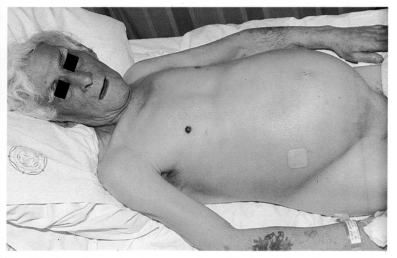

Fig. 139 Jaundice and ascites in a patient with chronic liver disease.

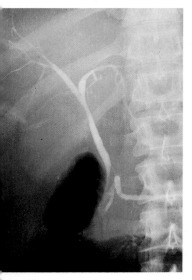

Fig. 140 A normal endoscopic cholangiogram.

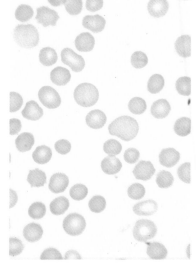

Fig. 141 Slide showing spherocytosis which may present with jaundice due to haemolysis.

Investigation

Biochemistry

Measurement of bilirubin, alkaline phosphatase and aspartate transaminase may help but may also give misleading results and by themselves are not able to classify jaundice. Urine testing of bilirubin and urobilinogen are of limited value. Gamma GT is very sensitive and may be an early sign of liver disease.

Proteins

Hypoalbuminaemia and clotting disorders which fail to respond to Vitamin K indicate impaired synthesis suggesting parenchymal disease.

Ultrasound

This will demonstrate whether the bile ducts are dilated favouring obstruction, or non-dilated favouring hepatocellular disease. The site of obstruction and its cause (e.g. gallstones) may be identified. Other features, (e.g. infiltration, fibrosis or fat) may also be seen.

Radiology

If ducts are dilated proceed either to endoscopic retrograde cholangiopancreatography (ERCP) or percutaneous transhepatic cholangiography (PTC) which should reveal the cause of obstruction.

Liver biopsy

If the ducts are normal and clotting allows then proceed to liver biopsy.

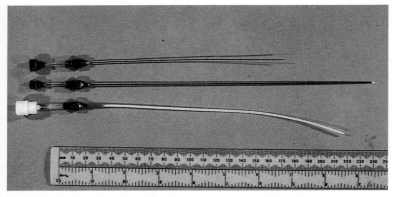

Fig. 142 A selection of needles for percutaneous cholangiography.

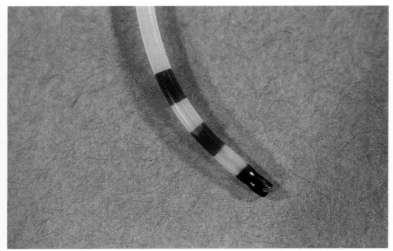

Fig. 143 The tip of an ERCP cannula.

Gilbert's syndrome
An isolated increase in serum bilirubin often found as an incidental finding occurring in 3–7% of normal individuals. Bilirubin may reach 103 µmol/l especially after a prolonged fast or in intercurrent infection. It is asymptomatic and should not require further investigation. Other congenital hyperbilirubinaemias are very rare and the more serious include Rotor, Dubin–Johnson and Crigler–Najjar syndromes.

Hepatitis

Viral
The term viral hepatitis usually refers to either hepatitis A, B or non-A, non-B hepatitis. However, other viruses including infectious mononucleosis, cytomegalovirus and herpes simplex may cause hepatitis.

Other
A number of bacteria, (e.g. leptospirosis), fungi and drugs can cause hepatitis. A mild hepatitis picture can also been seen in a number of systemic and infectious diseases and in heart failure.

Course of disease
Viral hepatitis may produce a spectrum of disease ranging from mild non-specific illness to severe fulminating fatal liver necrosis (fortunately it is very rare, i.e. seen in less than 1% of cases).

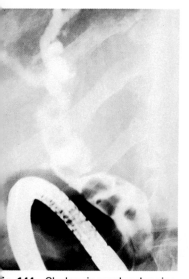

Fig. 144 Cholangiography showing multiple gall stones in a dilated biliary tree.

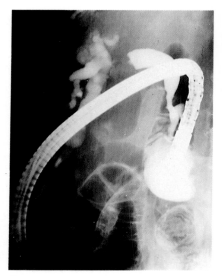

Fig. 145 Endoscopic cholangiography showing carcinoma of the bile duct.

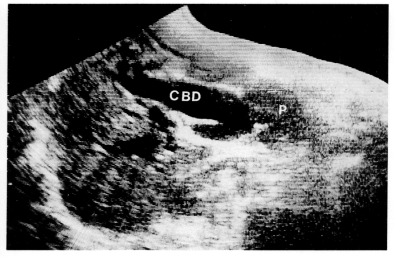

Fig. 146 Dilated common bile duct on ultrasound in obstructive jaundice.

| # Acute Hepatitis (1)

Hepatitis A

This has a short incubation period (21–35 days). It has a faecal–oral route of spread. It can be sporadic or epidemic and does not progress to chronic liver disease. It is diagnosed by finding HAV IgM antibody in serum indicating recent infection.

Hepatitis B

This has a longer incubation period (approximately 3 months). It is spread by parenteral contact with blood products by blood transfusion or by drug addicts sharing needles. Also there can be venereal spread, particularly by homosexuals. The most common method of spread world-wide is by mother to infant transmission perinatally. It occurs sporadically. Diagnosis is by finding HbsAg in serum. 'e' antigen suggests viral replication and infectivity. It may progress to carrier state or chronic hepatitis. Delta agent may cause superimposed hepatitis in known HbsAg-positive patients. Safe prophylactic active immunisation is now available.

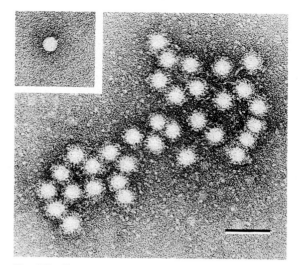

Fig. 147 Hepatitis A viral particle.

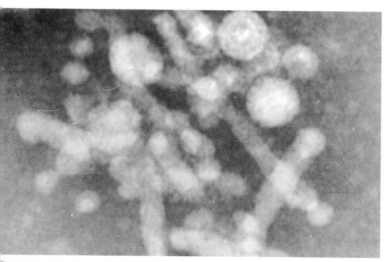

Fig. 148 EM of hepatitis B viral particle.

Non-A, Non-B

This is diagnosed by exclusion. There are several different viruses. They have intermediate incubation periods. Low grade hepatitis with progression to chronicity is common. Spread is as for hepatitis A or B.

Presentation

Presentation may be variable with symptoms of anorexia, nausea, fatigue, distaste for cigarettes, weight loss, fever, arthralgia, urticaria, jaundice, dark urine with pale stools, vasculitis, glomerulonephritis or hepatosplenomegaly.

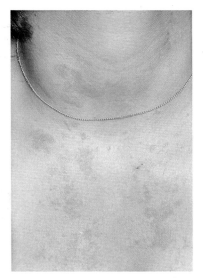

Fig. 149 Urticaria, an occasional prodromal feature of viral hepatitis.

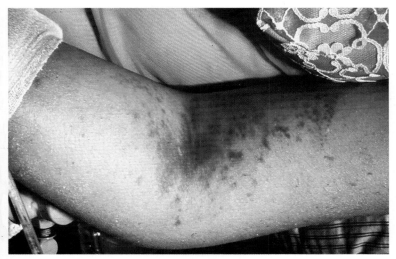

Fig. 150 Spontaneous bruising in severe hepatitis.

40 | Chronic Hepatitis

Definition
Chronic hepatitis indicates continued inflammation of the liver for more than 6 months. Liver biopsy is crucial for accurate diagnosis. It does not occur after hepatitis A.

Carrier state
An asymptomatic HbsAg-positive carrier state exists. There is a striking geographic variation : 0.1% in W Europe and the USA compared to 10% in SE Asia. The liver is often entirely normal. Patients are at longterm risk of developing chronic liver disease and hepatoma.

Chronic persistent hepatitis
This is a mild illness, often asymptomatic although mild non-specific symptoms are common. It does not progress to cirrhosis. A histological feature is that of normal architecture with a mononuclear (predominant lymphocytic) infiltrate in the portal tract.

Chronic active hepatitis
This is a more serious illness with a high probability of progressing to cirrhosis. Biopsies show piecemeal necrosis, parenchymal degeneration and regeneration progressing to distorted architecture and cirrhosis.

THE LIVER

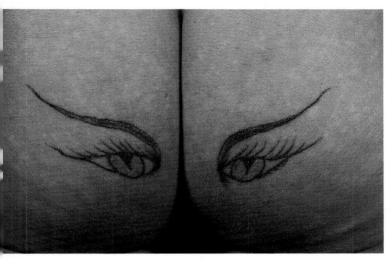

Fig. 151 Tattoos, a risk factor for hepatitis.

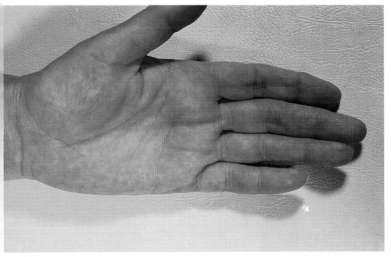

Fig. 152 Palmar erythema in acute hepatitis.

41 | Cirrhosis (1)

Definition

A diffuse histological process characterised by fibrosis and a conversion of normal architecture into structurally abnormal nodules. This incorporates cell death, disordered regeneration and fibrosis. Histologically it can be divided into micronodular or macronodular.

Micronodular

Small macroscopically indistinct nodules are seen in alcoholics, haemochromatosis, biliary obstruction and chronic active hepatitis.

Macronodular

Large often bulging nodules of varying size, often separated by broad fibrous bands, are seen in chronic hepatitis and as an end stage of almost any aetiology.

Symptoms

Symptoms are often non-specific but include general malaise, abdominal discomfort, loss of libido, jaundice, pruritus, fever, fluid retention, gastrointestinal haemorrhage, pigmentation, hepatosplenomegaly and incidental biochemical observation or with cutaneous stigmata of chronic liver disease.

THE LIVER

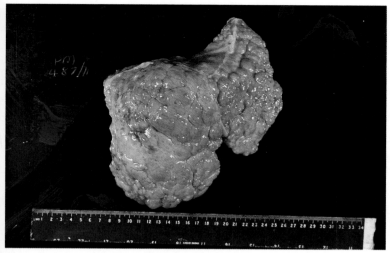

Fig. 153 Micronodular cirrhosis of the liver.

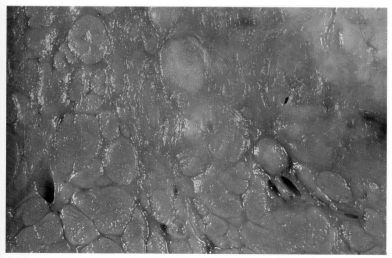

Fig. 154 Close-up of cirrhotic nodules on cut surface of liver.

41 | Cirrhosis (2)

Classification

Drugs and toxins	Alcohol and drugs including methotrexate and methyldopa.
Infections	Acute hepatitis, *Schistosoma japonica*.
Auto-immune	Primary biliary cirrhosis, chronic active hepatitis.
Metabolic	Wilson's disease, haemochromatosis, alpha$_1$ antitrypsin deficiency. Rarities include galactosaemia and porphyria.
Biliary obstruction	Sclerosing cholangitis, longstanding obstruction.
Vascular	Chronic right-sided heart failure, Budd—Chiari's syndrome, veno-occlusive disease, hereditary telangiectasia.
Infiltration	Sarcoid and amyloidosis.
Other	Intestinal bypass, Indian childhood cirrhosis.

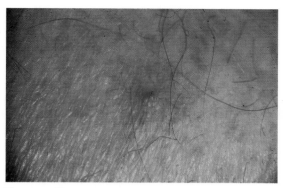

Fig. 155 Close-up of spider naevi.

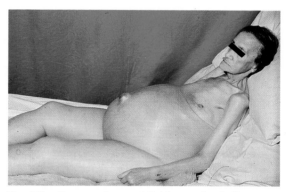

Fig. 156 Gross ascites and fluid retention in liver failure. Note the protruding umbilicus.

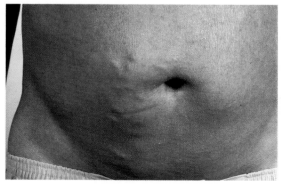

Fig. 157 Caput medusae.

Cirrhosis (3)

Clinical features

Hepatic failure

Hepatomegaly, low grade fever, bleeding tendency, faetor hepaticus, encephalopathy, water retention with ascites, susceptibility to infection, flapping tremor and parotid enlargement.

Cutaneous signs

White nails, palmar erythema, spider naevi, Dupuytren's contracture, finger clubbing.

Endocrine

Gynaecomastia, testicular atrophy and scanty body hair. In females, erratic menstruation and breast atrophy. Redistribution of body fat to trunk with skinny limbs (pseudo-Cushing's syndrome).

Portal hypertension

Splenomegaly, varices, caput medusa, GI bleeding and ascites.

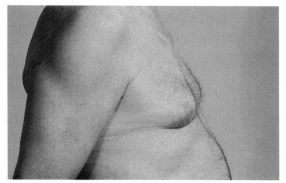

Fig. 158   Gynaecomastia.

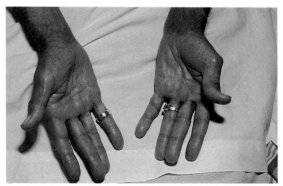

Fig. 159   Palmar erythema

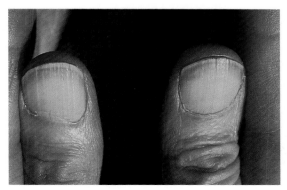

Fig. 160   Leukonychia.

42 | Haemochromatosis

Definition

Condition in which there is familial HLA-related parenchymal iron overloading. Iron is deposited in the liver, pancreas, testes, pituitary, adrenals and skin. It is clinically distinct from secondary iron overload state (haemosiderosis).

Aetiology

Autosomal recessive trait results in absorption of more iron than is necessary. Within families there is HLA association of the condition with certain phenotypes. Incidence is 1 in 500 for the homozygous state.

Presentation

Males outnumber females 10 to 1 (because of menstrual loss in females). Presentation is in the 5th to 6th decade with cirrhosis which has the notable additional features of slate grey pigmentation and diabetes (bronze diabetes). There is prominent testicular atrophy and hepatomegaly and it can be complicated in the longterm by hepatoma.

Diagnosis

Elevated serum iron, increased transferrin saturation and ferritin level. It always needs to be confirmed by liver biopsy. It is vital to screen family members of index cases.

Treatment

Venesection is the mainstay of treatment and will prevent progression of the cirrhosis. It is important to diagnose family members in the pre-cirrhotic phase.

THE LIVER

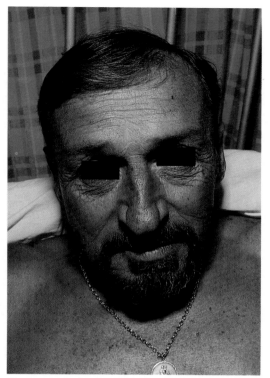

Fig. 161 Pigmentation in haemochromatosis.

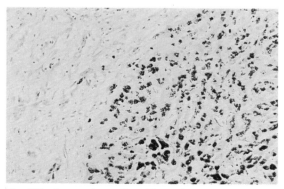

Fig. 162 Iron stain on liver biopsy in haemochromatosis showing Grade 4 iron overload.

43 | Wilson's Disease (hepatolenticular degeneration)

Definition

This is a fatal defect in the copper metabolism with reduced amounts of the copper-carrying protein (caeruloplasmin). Copper is deposited in the liver and brain and there is excess urine excretion.

Aetiology

An autosomal recessive with an incidence of about 1 in 30 000.

Presentation

The signs and symptoms of chronic liver disease are most common. It may present acutely with fluid retention and liver failure or more chronically with special features including haemolysis, Kayser—Fleischer rings and renal tubular acidosis. It may present with neurological symptoms including rigidity, coarse tremor and intellectual deterioration.

Diagnosis

Increased urinary copper levels, reduced serum caeruloplasmin and increased non-caeruloplasmin serum copper. Liver biopsy shows excessive hepatic copper deposition and is often required to confirm diagnosis.

Treatment

Chelating agents, usually D-penicillamine. It is important to diagnose the disease early and therefore family members of index cases should be carefully screened.

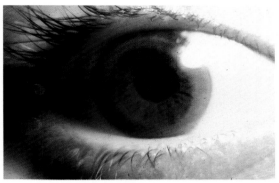

Fig. 163 Kayser–Fleischer rings.

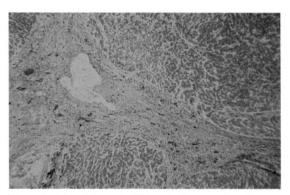

Fig. 164 Liver biopsy in Wilson's disease showing excess copper.

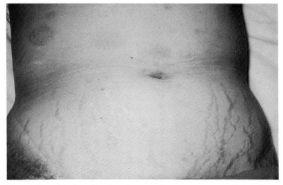

Fig. 165 Abdominal striae and spontaneous bruising in a patient with Wilson's disease.

44 | Primary Biliary Cirrhosis

Definition

A progressive immunologically mediated liver disease, characterised by progressive intrahepatic cholestasis and cirrhosis.

Presentation

Primarily a disease of women (90%). Early symptoms of pruritus followed by signs and symptoms of chronic liver disease. Particular features include xanthelasma, finger clubbing and deep pigmentation.

Investigations

Progressive cholestatic jaundice leading to cirrhosis. Antimitochondrial antibody is positive in 98%. Diagnosis is confirmed by liver biopsy.

Disease course

Slow but relentless progression. Associated conditions include scleroderma, Sjögren's syndrome, renal tubular acidosis and other connective tissue diseases.

Treatment

Penicillamine and azathioprine have been shown to be of benefit but are associated with considerable side-effects. Liver transplant can be carried out in suitable cases. Cholestyramine may ease pruritus and vitamin replacement is important. Corticosteroids are not indicated and they may result in rapid bone demineralisation.

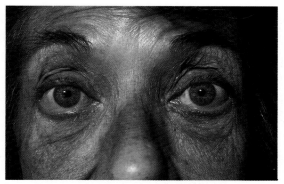

Fig. 166 Pigmented jaundice in primary biliary cirrhosis.

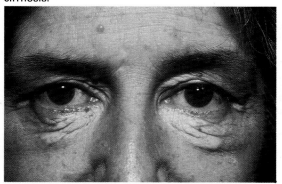

Fig. 167 Severe xanthelasmata in primary biliary cirrhosis.

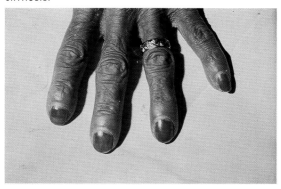

Fig. 168 Severe finger clubbing and pigmentation in primary biliary cirrhosis.

45 | Chronic Active Hepatitis (lupoid hepatitis) of Unknown Aetiology

Terminology

This excludes those conditions which also produce histological chronic active hepatitis, (i.e. chronic HbsAg-associated, drug induced, alpha$_1$ antitrypsin deficiency and Wilson's disease).

Presentation

It primarily affects young women. There are features of acute or chronic liver disease particularly general malaise, sometimes butterfly rash and other features of systemic lupus erythematosus (SLE).

Investigations

Biochemistry reveals a hepatocellular picture. Gammaglobulins non-specifically increased, particularly IgG. Antinuclear factor antibody is positive with positive LE cells. Diagnosis is confirmed by liver biopsy.

Disease course

Classically it shows excellent clinical response to corticosteroids and azathioprine. Associated conditions include Sjögren's syndrome, renal tubular acidosis, ulcerative colitis, arthropathy, connective tissue diseases and haemolytic anaemia.

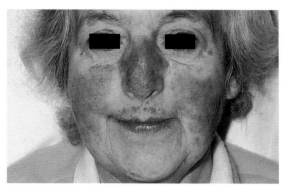

Fig. 169 Butterfly rash in chronic active hepatitis.

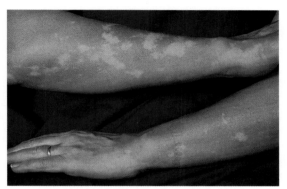

Fig. 170 Vitiligo in chronic active hepatitis.

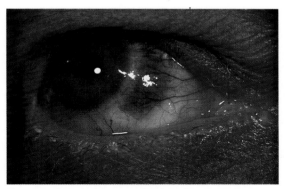

Fig. 171 Episcleritis complicating chronic active hepatitis.

Cryptogenic

A large proportion of patients with end-stage cirrhosis do not fall into any of the diagnostic groups described above.

Alpha₁ antitrypsin deficiency

Homozygous disease occurs in 1 in 1500 of the population, presenting with neonatal jaundice and chronic liver disease in early adult life. Heterozygous disease (1 in 20) may be asymptomatic or present in later life with established cirrhosis. Diagnosis is confirmed by finding PAS-positive globules on liver biopsy and by phenotyping. Serum alpha₁ antitrypsin levels alone may be misleading.

Cardiac cirrhosis

Cirrhosis may complicate severe and prolonged right heart failure. Treatment is that of the underlying heart disease.

Sarcoid

Cirrhosis may be encountered in late stage sarcoidosis.

Hydatid disease

Ova of *Taenia echinococcus* multiply in the liver and produce daughter cysts. It may present with progressive jaundice or remain localised.

Schistosomiasis

A cause of progressive cirrhosis in endemic regions.

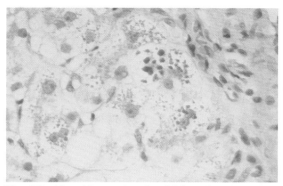

Fig. 172 Liver biopsy showing PAS-positive globules in alpha₁ anti-trypsin deficiency.

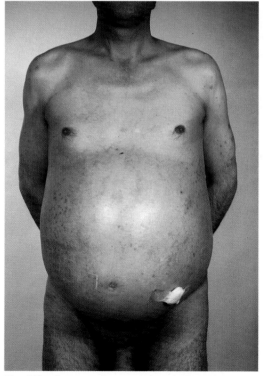

Fig. 173 Gross ascites and chronic liver disease with evidence of a recent diagnostic tap.

47 | Alcoholic Liver Disease

Prevalence

This is the commonest cause of liver disease in Western civilisation and is the fifth most common cause of death in men aged 25–64. It is directly related to the amount, but not type, of alcohol consumption. The exact mechanism of toxicity is unknown. Safe alcohol intake is 40g per day in men and less in women.

Progression of disease

Presentation may occur after several years of asymptomatic heavy drinking. The sequence of disease varies from fatty liver, alcoholic hepatitis to established cirrhosis. The presentation may be medical or psychological and may be at any stage.

Fatty liver

Fat accumulation in the liver, which may also be seen in obesity, diabetes, starvation and some systemic diseases is reversible on discontinuing alcohol.

Alcoholic hepatitis

This is more sinister and if drinking continues will eventually progress to cirrhosis. Histological features include inflammatory infiltrate and Mallory bodies.

Cirrhosis

It is usually micronodular in the early stages.

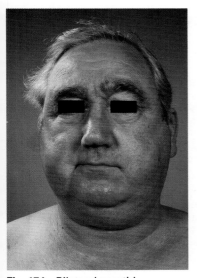

Fig. 174 Bilateral parotid enlargement in patient with alcoholic liver disease.

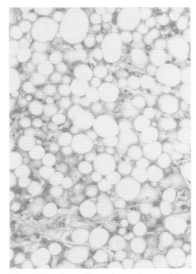

Fig. 175 Fatty liver in patient with alcoholic liver disease.

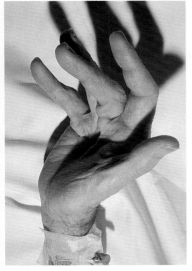

Fig. 176 Dupuytren's contracture in patient with liver disease.

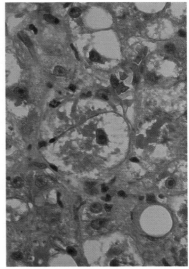

Fig. 177 Mallory body on liver biopsy in patient with alcoholic hepatitis.

Portal Hypertension (1)

Causes

1. *Pre-sinusoidal*: portal vein obstruction either extrahepatitic (thrombosis or malignancy) or intrahepatic (congenital hepatic fibrosis, schistosomiasis).
2. *Sinusoidal*: cirrhosis is by far the most common cause.
3. *Post-sinusoidal*: hepatic vein obstruction

Sites of anastomosis

1. Gastro-oesophageal veins.
2. Spleno-oesophageal and diaphragmatic or peritoneal anastomosis.
3. Umbilical vein.
4. Superior surface of liver and diaphragm.
5. Mesenteric and haemorrhoidal veins.

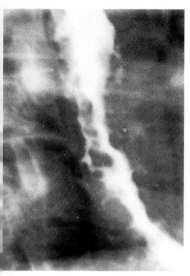

Fig. 178 Barium swallow showing varices.

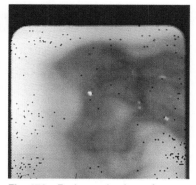

Fig. 179 Endoscopic view of varices.

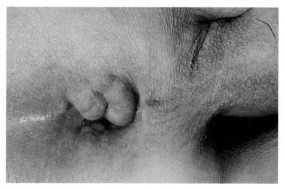

Fig. 180 Anal varices.

48 | Portal Hypertension (2)

Presentation

Severe GI bleeding with oesophageal or anal varices, gross splenomegaly, portal systemic encephalopathy. Blood flow in caput medusa is away from the umbilicus.

Treatment

Bleeding temporarily stopped by vasoconstriction with Vasopressin or balloon tamponade. Endoscopic sclerotherapy has largely replaced the portal-systemic shunt operation as the treatment of choice because of unacceptable complications of the latter.

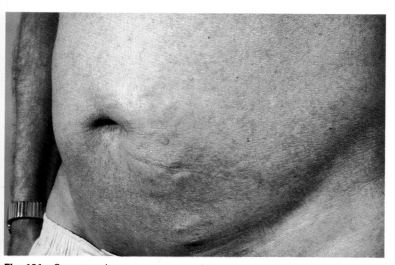

Fig. 181 Caput medusae.

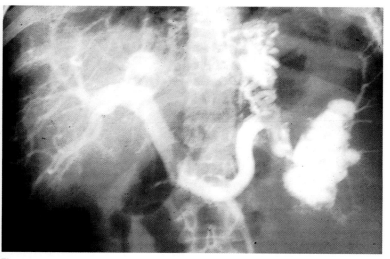

Fig. 182 Splenoportogram showing oesophageal varices.

49 | Budd–Chiari Syndrome

Aetiology

A very rare syndrome which results from thrombotic occlusion of the hepatic vein. It is associated with neoplasia, polycythaemia and the contraceptive Pill.

Presentation

Acute onset of abdominal pain, tender hepatomegaly, ascites and acute hepatic necrosis. One-third present chronically.

Diagnosis

Ultrasound shows gross venous distension and radio-isotope liver scan shows the specific feature of maximum uptake in the caudate lobe in some patients. Diagnosis may be confirmed by liver biopsy or arteriography.

Treatment

Treatment is symptomatic or by liver transplantion if possible.

Congenital hepatic fibrosis

Pathology

Bands of fibrous tissue join all portal tracts.

Presentation

Portal hypertension. Liver function remains well preserved.

THE LIVER

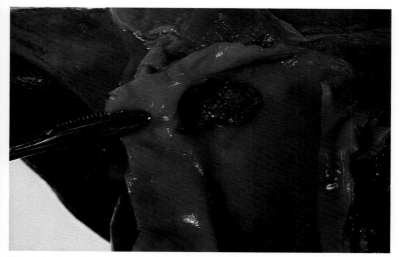

Fig. 183 Surgical specimen showing thrombus in the left hepatic vein in Budd—Chiari syndrome.

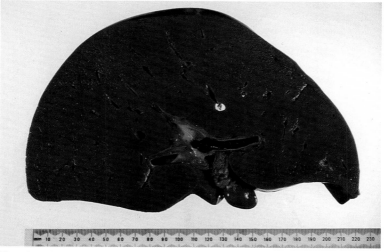

Fig. 184 Portal vein thrombus.

50 | Liver Abscess

Classification
Pyogenic or amoebic. It may be single or multiple. It may occur spontaneously or may complicate intra-abdominal sepsis, hepatic trauma or ascending cholangitis. Common organisms include gram-negative organisms and streptococcal species.

Presentation
Abdominal pain, swinging pyrexia, night sweats, anorexia, weight loss and local tenderness.

Diagnosis
Ultrasound has greatly simplified diagnosis. CT scanning may also help but aspiration is diagnostic and enables direct microscopy and culture of organisms. An amoebic abscess typically contains 'anchovy sauce'-like fluid.

Treatment
Non-operative drainage with repeated needle aspiration or catheter insertion together with relevant antibiotics has replaced surgical drainage as first-line treatment.

Differential diagnosis
This includes necrotic solid tumours and polycystic disease of the liver.

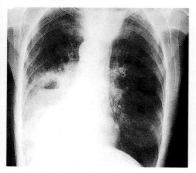

Fig. 185 Chest X-ray in patient with liver abscess showing a raised right hemidiaphragm with fluid level.

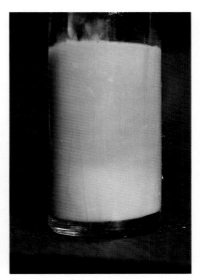

Fig. 186 'Anchovy sauce' aspirated from an amoebic abscess.

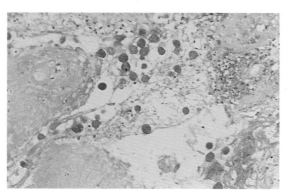

Fig. 187 PAS stain of amoebic pus.

51 | Liver Failure

Acute fulmonant

This may result from viral hepatitis, paracetamol overdose, halothane or other toxins.

Decompensated chronic liver disease

This is due to GI haemorrhage, septicaemia, spontaneous bacterial peritonitis, hepatoma and inappropriate drug treatment, e.g. narcotics and diuretics.

Presentation

Confusion, apraxia, behaviour disturbance, asterixis, pre-coma and coma.

Treatment

Treatment is mainly supportive. Lactulose or neomycin will reduce the protein load in the gut. Intravenous dextrose will prevent hypoglycaemia. Antibiotics and vitamin replacements can be given as required.

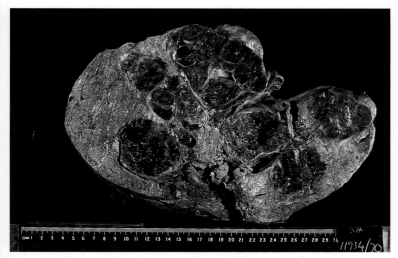

Fig. 188 Hepatoma in post mortem liver specimen.

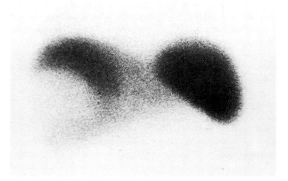

Fig. 189 Liver scan showing solitary filling defect in patient with hepatoma.

52 | Hepatoma

Incidence

There is a wide geographic variation. It is rare in the UK and USA but common in countries with a high carrier rate of HbsAg, e.g. Taiwan and parts of Africa. There is a strong association with HbSag infection due to integration of viral DNA into host hepatocytes. It is also encountered in patients with longstanding cirrhosis and after aflotoxin ingestion.

Presentation

Sudden worsening of established chronic liver disease or abdominal pain, anorexia and weight loss. There can be symptoms of secondary spread to lungs or bone.

Diagnosis

This is often associated with a very high level of alpha fetoprotein in the serum. Ultrasound, CT scan and liver biopsy are confirmatory.

Treatment

Prognosis is poor. Surgical excision is the only chance of cure and success depends on the extent of the disease. Chemotherapy and therapeutic embolisation may palliate. Hepatitis B prophylactic vaccination may have a preventive role in future.

Differential diagnosis

This includes primary tumour of the bile duct (cholangiocarcinoma).

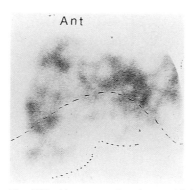

Fig. 190 Liver scan showing multiple metastases.

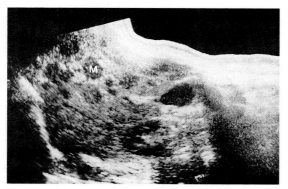

Fig. 191 Ultrasound of the liver showing metastases.

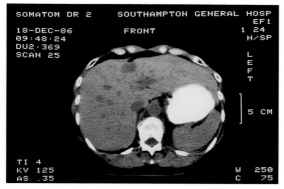

Fig. 192 CT showing multiple liver metastases.

53 | Sclerosing Cholangitis

Definition

There is progressive destruction of the intra-or extra- hepatic biliary system. Predominantly it affects young men. It is usually seen in association with ulcerative colitis, also Crohn's colitis, sclerosing mediastinitis and retroperitoneal fibrosis.

Presentation

There is usually progressive biochemical evidence of cholestasis but symptoms include pruritus and general malaise. Natural history of the disease varies but the disease course may be very long and fluctuating.

Diagnosis

ERCP is diagnostic. Liver biopsy may not be conclusive but it may show narrowed bile ductules surrounded by diffuse fibrous rings with features of large bile duct obstruction.

Treatment

There is no specific treatment. Endoscopic dilatation of the stricture may help. Steroids are of unproven benefit. Liver transplantation can be in selected cases.

Differential diagnosis

Gallstone-associated strictures and primary cholangiocarcinomas must be excluded. It may be confused with Caroli disease which is a rare condition involving intrahepatic dilatation of the bile ducts.

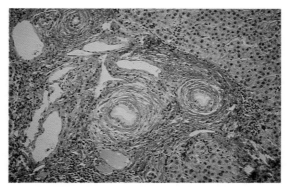

Fig. 193 Histology of sclerosing cholangitis showing multiple 'onion rings'.

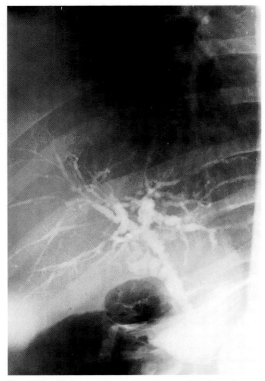

Fig. 194 Endoscopic cholangiography showing beading and irregularities in sclerosing cholangitis.

54 | Gallstones

Cause

Pigment stones occur in chronic haemolytic anaemias. Cholesterol stones occur due to supersaturation of bile salts. The latter are found with increasing age traditionally in the 'fat, female, fair and forty' patient group.

Presentation

Varied. Right hypochondrial pain and flatulence are most common but it may present with acute cholecystitis, empyema of the gall bladder or obstructive jaundice due to a stone in the common bile duct.

Treatment

Silent gallstones may not require treatment. Medical treatment with dissolution therapy is disappointing and most experts still recommend surgical intervention. Stones in the common bile duct can be treated by endoscopic sphincterotomy. Lithotripsy is a potential non-surgical treatment.

Complications

Complications include obstructive jaundice, pancreatitis, ascending cholangitis. Gas in the biliary tree indicates either infection with gas-forming organisms or biliary fistula due to passage of a stone.

Diagnosis

Plain abdominal X-ray may reveal a calcified stone. Otherwise diagnosis is by oral cholecystogram or ultrasound.

THE LIVER

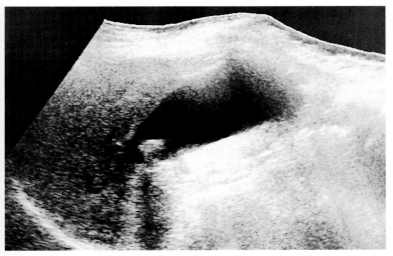

Fig. 195 Ultrasound showing gallstone in dilated gall bladder.

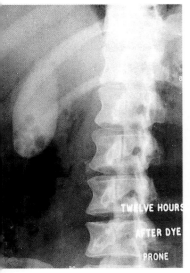

Fig. 196 Gallstones shown on oral cholangiogram.

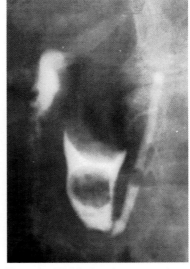

Fig. 197 ERCP showing stones in dilated biliary tree.

Index